LUCKY STROKE

Subarachnoid Hemorrhage
Thoughts of a Survivor

Glenn M. Peach

G. M. PEACH

Cover design by Lisa Engelbach

ISBN-10: 1514307634
ISBN-13: 978-1514307632

This is dedicated to the ones I love.
You give me the love and encouragement, the optimism
and patience, and the certainty that luck is all around us.

G. M. PEACH

CONTENTS

G. M. PEACH

Out of the sane, silent, beauteous
miracles that envelope and fuse
me –trees, water, grass, sunlight,
and early frost –the one I am
looking at most to-day is the sky.

Walt Whitman (1882)
Specimen Days and Collect

G. M. PEACH

Preface

It is not so important for this story to explain what I, an American, was doing in Germany when my brain decided to have a stroke. Let it suffice to say, that our country sends its young men off to distant lands at a vulnerable age. Some find reasons to stay or to return to those places later in their lives. So it was for me.

Stroke is an illness that could happen to anyone, anytime, anywhere. My own stroke was miraculously kind to me and it took me on a journey to seek explanations for what happens in the bodies and the minds of the victims of stroke. The experiences described here are my own. They may be similar to hundreds of thousands of other people who never get the chance to describe them to others. Some of the other information presented is widely accessible from numerous online sources.

There are many different varieties and intensities of

stroke, but the symptoms and initial hours and days and weeks of treatment take on a similar pattern for all those who survive the initial attack, whether male or female, old or young. It is important to know the warning signs of stroke and the proper response to take when it strikes. Other sources such as the website of the National Stroke Association (www.stroke.org) offer more comprehensive information.

The aim of all treatment methods is to restore, improve, and maintain good health. It is no different for the victims of a stroke. Those who survive are already among the lucky ones, for stroke is the third most common killer in America behind heart disease and cancer. Then, if their luck holds, they enter a treatment process that gives them the encouragement and the patience and the courage to heal themselves. Then, if they are really lucky, they learn something new about themselves and their world.

"Who am I tellin' you?"

JJ Cale, song lyrics

G. M. PEACH

CHAPTER 1

An innocent man!

OK, so I was just dead lucky. That's what the doctors said for lack of any other explanation. How strange that something so common and deadly still leaves the doctors wondering. Maybe that's because most of the victims are unable to talk about it afterwards. Even those who witness it are also, at least temporarily, paralyzed. As common as it is, it is very personal and private and comes in so many shocking forms. We have all heard about this kind of thing, but few of us really know what is happening or what action to take. What happens when you have a stroke? This is an account of a particularly deadly form of stroke – a red stroke – a subarachnoid hemorrhage – my stroke.

Strokes happen to people all the time, but always to the other guy, right? You probably know someone in your extended family, the neighborhood, your circle of friends, celebrities, etc. But they are outside of your immediate range of contact, too far away, or it is too scary or too sad - a subject too easily avoided. You never think it will happen to you. Peter Gabriel could be referring to it in *Don't Give Up:*

> *"Though I saw it all around, never thought I could be affected, thought that we'd be the last to go, it is so strange the way things turn."*

Am I lucky? Hard to say, but that is the explanation so often used when no other is available. I certainly had my share of luck growing up in what was the great post-war middle class, I had never seen misfortune. Born and raised under the New England work ethic, I had been taught to think people make their own luck. Life was decided by hard work, cooperation, and pragmatic decisions and then a benevolent God rewards you. Maybe that is how it is. Someone else once said "Luck is recognizing opportunity as it passes by and taking advantage of it." That works for me too. I had been lucky all my life, shielded from the misfortunes or "unpleasantness" encountered by others. Bad stuff just didn't happen in my world. My world didn't include major illnesses. I could rely on that. It is sort of like being immunized by luck when it is always there. There is no need to fear the future, no anxieties about work. No matter what comes at you, something inside tells you that it will be alright. There can be no other option. As you read this you may be thinking "what a privileged jerk" or, rather I hope you will recognize something of yourself here too, for many times, it is true that you make your own luck. If you are affected by stroke, what you will need is luck, like I needed it, to pull you out of harm's way!

Some of you baby boomers will remember Rod Serling's weekly, black and white TV show which opened with a distinctive male voice saying: "Picture a man, going on a journey, beyond sight and sound. He has entered *"the twilight zone."* Those stories were about average people in extraordinary situations. Each episode was a search for some emotional truth and the main character was either dead or he returned with a better understanding of himself. The story endings were a lot like the ending to this story. That's right, in this episode, I return. I am alive and well and I have a better understanding of my world and myself. I am one of the lucky few who can tell this, no, my story.

But why am I telling you this? Who am I to tell you? Why bother with what I have to say? We don't know each other and I have no public image and I am not pitching a cause like so many of the books written on this subject do. I am someone like you or your loved one, or a close relative, a neighbor, or perhaps, your patient. Placing what is said into the context of who says it usually helps in understanding the message.

Before this happened, I had no idea about stroke or the

many people affected in some way by stroke. I was "*An Innocent Man*" like the one in Billy Joel's song:

> *"I know you don't want to hear what I say. I know you're gonna keep turning away. But I've been there and if I can survive, I can keep you alive."*

Now, I have seen the things that happen after a diagnosis of "stroke." This book is simply my account of all the stops along a journey that every stroke victim takes. From the start, I know some of the worries and concerns you have. Towards the middle of the story, I am frustrated by the doctor's use of the mysterious term "self-healing" and I search for a more technical explanation. I share some of the research done to help in my own understanding of how I survived undamaged. But, mostly this book is a compilation of memories and now that it is over, finally, I stop crying.

Like one of Rod Serling's plots, stroke recovery demands the victim deal with an emotional event. This illness doesn't stop when you survive the first twenty four hours, or when you leave the hospital, or even when the rehab phase is over. For some unfortunate victims who survive, it may never be over. Three quarters of a million Americans will take this trip this year. It will happen to hundreds of thousands more too, in places like Britain, Russia, Japan, and Germany. Data from the developed countries shows that it will happen 15 million times each year and will result in 5 million deaths and an additional 5 million patients living with permanent dependency.

Another 5 million will have varying levels of hardship.

Am I healthy today because I was lucky or maybe I was lucky just because I am healthy? Experiencing and surviving a deadly stroke made me wonder about things like that. Any way you phrase it, stroke is nothing if not an emotional journey – for the victim and many others.

It happened to me without any warning and immediately took me out of the realm of familiar experience. I was having a stroke, a brain bleed. My journey to the twilight zone had begun. There came a momentary strange feeling, not necessarily painful, just one that you can perceive as being different; a discomfort, sort of an inner void, as if the senses to the outside were being shut down; the outside world slowly becoming irrelevant, it has started. Something has taken over your attention and you know, no, you feel there is a problem. You feel there is something wrong inside your head but you are not sure what it is.

Maybe someone you care for has entered the twilight zone and is making the journey right now. I can't say how the illness will affect them. No one can do that. I can only share the tests, treatments, feelings, places, thoughts, and lucky encounters – from the first onset of symptoms to the return home and the days, months and years thereafter. This story is written in chronological order so you can prepare for what is coming next on the new and disconcerting journey brought on by stroke. Above all else, it tells you that you're on your own, but you are not alone.

You don't always notice it; the luck I mean, because you think you have it all under control, but luck is also there, waiting to help when you need it. Looking back now, it must have been with me all through my life, always somewhere in the background. According to my Mom, her doctor told her 57 years ago that I was expected to be a stillborn birth. My Dad drove her to the big city hospital of Providence, RI where, as luck would have it, she gave birth to a healthy baby boy. I had a lucky childhood, spending the summers on Cape Cod, playing barefoot on sandy roads and fishing off the jetties; learning how to hammer nails from my grandfather and how to sail from my older brother.

The direction my life took after graduating from high school in 1971 is another example of luck checking-in on me in unexpected ways. The national military draft back then was based on your birthday and mine drew the number 33. If you were a male born on a day with a number from 1 to 150, you would be called up to serve your country and most likely be shipped off to Viet Nam, a place not too many could find on a map even now. That was a time when many young Americans were burning their draft cards in protest and moving to Canada rather than fight in an unjust war. In 1971, ordinary citizens even broke into the FBI office in Media, Pennsylvania to expose illegal government surveillance programs directed at anti-war protestors. It was also a time when college was the most widely used legal deferment to avoid having to report immediately for those called up for enlistment. So, having the opportunities of the white middle class, I went off to college thinking no war can last another four years and left politics to others more informed than I was. Of course, no one knew it back then, but by the time I was to graduate, the war and the draft would be over. No more draft numbers would ever be called to serve. The all-volunteer military would be advertised with exciting TV ads and women would be allowed into the service academies.

But luck wasn't taking any chances with me: On one of his business trips, my Dad, who was a salesman for a jewelry manufacturer stepped into a hotel elevator with Mel Pender, the fastest man in the world in 1960 and then the coach of the West Point track team. A short time later, an application for the United States Military Academy at West Point, New York arrived in the mail for me. I had never thought about applying there even when the draft was looming. So, I checked it out and decided to leave college and become an officer. The deadline for applications had passed, but my congresswoman somehow managed a waiver and my application was accepted. After graduation, I was a second lieutenant in the US Army on my way to Germany. Luck followed me and placed a cute, brown-eyed Bavarian girl in my path. Cupid got off two lucky shots and we have been sharing our lives together ever since. She became the mother of my two children and the family has been healthy and happy and lucky together all these years.

I have enjoyed opportunities that most people never get. In the Army, for example, I managed to stay pretty fit with 5-mile runs and physical training at 6:00 o'clock every morning all year round. I got to parachute out of Belgian army balloons, fly in an F16B and experience "9-Gs" with a top gun pilot. I am also very grateful to some extraordinary soldiers, one of whom, years later, was in a position to save my career from a bad decision in a broken down system – another lucky constellation at the right moment. Each turning point in my life was "grazed" by the presence of what we can call "luck." But, the turning point remembered in this book is in a class all by itself and gets an intentional spelling change: I had been "graced."

Answers, like strokes, are individual and each survivor must deal with the present and hope for the future using all the powers at their disposal. Some may find the courage to reprogram their goals for the future, but if it simply helps to bring some understanding and hope to those forced to experience a frightening situation, whether the victim or the caregiver, like it did for me, this book will have served its purpose.

Let's start at the beginning.

"Luck often enough, will save
a man, if his courage hold."

Buliwyf, *in*
The 13th Warrior

G. M. PEACH

CHAPTER 2

What happened?

Traffic was flowing smoothly at over 90 miles per hour on the German *Autobahn*. I had just driven the 40 miles to the campus of the University of Saarland to meet with a small class of talented language students. The scene seemed so ordinary, so harmless. They were all seated at their desks waiting for me to explain the difference in the proper usage of *that* and *which* or any of the other peculiarities that occur with some regularity in the English language. The class meets every Wednesday at 11:30 in the morning and I show up to teach them how to translate technical German texts into English so that laymen can read and understand. This is what I do now, my first job after a very varied Army life. The class was scheduled to last until 1:30 p.m., but on this sunny Wednesday, at about 12:15, something was happening well below the surface – something beyond the wildest imagination of a healthy, happy, active person.

No, it was not a teenager dressed in black that had entered the room with an automatic weapon. What happened was much more sinister than that because it is invisible and there is no warning and it is meant for you and you alone. A very strange feeling, a very, very, strange feeling came over me. My reaction was immediate. It was a sensation that left no doubt. Not wanting to interrupt classroom decorum and show my discomfort in front of the students, I excused myself to go to a nearby men's room. There, I splashed cold water on my face and brow. Then, feeling a bit light headed and nauseous, I turned to move toward the toilets. I took two steps in that direction and that is when the excruciating headache forced me down onto the floor – a perspective of a public toilet that few people ever get. At first, I thought lying down might help it to go away. But, it didn't. The pain was building as I lay there on my back unable (unwilling?) to move. I knew that something quite out of the ordinary was happening to me and that if I didn't get up right away, I may never get up. I said to myself, "I am not going to stay here on the floor to die in a public toilet." I forced myself back up onto my feet and moved cautiously back to the classroom.

As fast as it arrived, the pain seemed to be slowing time itself down. In the doorway, I said, "Sorry, I have never felt like this before. I am afraid class is dismissed." I gathered up my materials and walked on shaky legs down the stairs to my car, leaving the students in their seats with questioning looks on their faces. No more than 10 minutes had elapsed.

I just sat in the car, thinking and willing the pain away. I discovered that when I pushed with my fingers on the spot at the lower back side of my skull where the pain seemed to be the greatest, it would temporarily subside – at least, this is what I was telling myself. I did this in a state of lowered consciousness for what I thought was 10-15 minutes, but when I looked at my watch, over an hour had passed. I called my wife on the mobile phone to tell her that something was wrong. She wanted to drive to the university to get me, but I said that is too complicated and it would take too long. After we hung up, I said to myself, "I need something now: *gotta get myself to a hospital.*" Instinctively, I knew time was going to be important. I figured I was my own fastest option. So I started the engine of my BMW and headed back to the German *Autobahn,* knowing the drive would take about half an hour. I still had no idea what was happening to me. I still had control over my hands and legs. Some stroke victims are unaware of the symptoms that others can perceive when they see or hear the victim – the irregularities in the face, arms, and speech. In my case, it was just the laming power of the pain in my head.

Once underway, I didn't want to stop for fear that I would not have the will to resume driving, but the pain in my head and the stiffness in my neck were unbearable and getting to be more constant. I pulled into a rest area along the way to get things back under control, but didn't stay parked there for long. Things were not getting any better so I grit my teeth together and told myself to move on and get help. "*Just a bit further,*" I said to myself. When the exit for the Landstuhl Regional Medical Center appeared, it was a welcome site. It is the largest American military hospital outside the continental United States, with about 2,800 employees. In recent years, it has been busy treating soldiers and photo journalists wounded in Iraq and Afghanistan. It is my health insurance, provided to me in my employment contract for serving all over the world in the US military for twenty years.

When I finally arrived at LRMC, I was *lucky* enough to find a parking spot very close to the ER entrance – the first of many miracles (if we don't count my surviving the German autobahn). I walked gingerly across the road and through the security check point. The automatic doors opened for me and I approached the admissions desk. The attendant seemed to respond much faster this time than I was accustomed to from my previous visits there. After straining to give a description of my problem while leaning on the check-in counter with my head down, I was asked if I was in pain. I have always had a problem when asked to rate my pain on a scale of 1 to 10. Pain is always personal and emotional. The military culture values stoicism. We are inclined to parade our toughness when face-to-face with pain. Here numbers take the place of words. Rate my pain in relation to what? Which one is a 6, a 7? Is my 3 your 5? Is Bob's 9, Betty's 2? Can anyone really feel a 10, or is it a concept for something unbearable. Do you expire after a 10? This routine scale of pain by the numbers seems a bit ambiguous at best. When I answered "11" she asked, "Would you say it was the worst headache of your life?" I got out the word "Yes!" A wheelchair appeared out of nowhere and I was on my way to the CT scanner. A CT scan uses x-rays; an MRI uses magnetic resonance and takes a lot longer to perform. I remember the wind in my face from the pace the attendant was pushing me.

The technician slid me into that cream colored tube and made some pictures of my brain. I shut my eyes. As soon as I was wheeled back into the ER, it became obvious that the test had seen something. Immediately, a stretcher arrived and I was somehow assisted out of my clothes and into the hospital gown, but not before I slipped my mobile phone out of my pocket and dialed my wife's office number. Her boss answered the phone on her desk and I got off the short message, "Tell her I am at Landstuhl and they are going to operate." It was a pretty insensitive message to leave, but I didn't have the strength or the time for a longer conversation.

I was placed on a gurney for transport. Two medics were searching my hands and arms for a suitable spot for the IV needle as the doctor appeared at my side and asked me to make a ring with my thumb and forefinger which he tried to pull apart. Then I showed him my teeth and puffed out my cheeks as he requested me to do. He seemed satisfied. "You have had a brain hemorrhage. We are not equipped to handle it here. We have made arrangements for you to go to a stroke unit."

Things were fuzzy at that point, but thanks to the quick actions of the ER team that day, I was properly diagnosed and loaded onto a stretcher for the transport to Homburg University Clinic. The doctor gave me two of the biggest capsules I had ever seen to swallow and the IV tubes were sending something into my arm - all for the purpose of stopping what was happening in my head.

I do not know how my wife managed it, but there she was. Her face appeared at the end of the stretcher while I waited those few minutes for the ambulance to arrive. She must have set a new, land speed record. I was so relieved to see her there, no matter what was to happen next. She was being briefed by the ER doctors, one of whom was a neurosurgeon. He had just told her that most of the people diagnosed as I had been are dead before the receptionist can ask the question: "Would you say it is the worst headache of your life?" I could see the fear and concern in my wife's eyes. But I knew then that everything would be alright. I smiled to give her some of my confidence. Together we would master this new situation just as we had mastered so many of life's other challenges – with a little luck. The German ambulance crew loaded me into the ambulance with my wife riding shotgun up front.

The ride to the University Clinic was uneventful. I was drifting blissfully along in that state of lowered consciousness, aware of when the driver turned on the siren and able to see through the back window. I was familiar with this route and knew the landmarks. Everyone can use a little humor in their high stress jobs. An attendant was seated somewhere behind me just out of sight and had not moved or said a word the entire time. Shortly after the ambulance took the final turn off the *Autobahn,* I said to him, "Hey, wake up. We are almost there!" No response. I did not know he was actually the emergency doctor and that he had been carefully monitoring me the whole time. Everyone knows *you just don't speak to a German doctor that way,* especially when he is trying to keep you alive. But, he took it in good stride and reported to the clinic's intensive care station that I had retained consciousness and was making jokes along the way. I know how very fortunate I was at that point to still be able to do that.

Since then, I have learned that time is very critical in treating stroke. The specialists say "time is brain." So far in this journey, maybe I was the only one who had wasted any time. Don't take the same risk. Learn the indicators of each kind of stroke and call the emergency number right away at the first sign of a stroke.

G. M. PEACH

"Scientists will save us all."

Johnny Gunther, *in*
Death Be Not Proud

G. M. PEACH

CHAPTER 3

The end of the English language

A what? Where the hell did that come from? That is a question that troubled me for a long time. Strokes are for the elderly, something that leaves them with slurred speech and in need of a walker. I had other plans like celebrating my 57th birthday in a few days. How could a stroke happen to me now? My son was about to make me a grandfather in a few weeks. My daughter wanted my help with a business power point presentation. I was way too young for this. I had suffered a subarachnoid hemorrhage (SAH), a brain bleed, one of the two forms of red stroke. The other is called ICH, or intracerebral hemorrhage. SAH is a medical emergency and usually leads to death or severe disability even when recognized and treated at an early stage. The German language has a way with military and medical terms. I didn't know it then, but I soon learned that what I had experienced was called in German appropriately, a "*Vernichtungskopfweh.*" It is a word that means annihilation or obliteration.

A stroke can happen at any age: only 30 percent of the victims are under the age of 65. The statistics for strokes are grim at best, and very often conflicting. In the United States alone, more than 780,000 people per year suffer a stroke and nearly 160,000 of them will die immediately as a result. The majority suffer what is called "ischemic stroke" or white stroke, where blood is blocked from getting to the brain. However, about 12 percent of the total is "hemorrhagic stroke" or red stroke, caused when too much blood collects in or around the brain. In addition to the pressure building on the cells in the area of the bleeding, the flow of blood is interrupted and oxygen rich blood fails to reach the intended brain tissue.

Subarachnoid hemorrhage (SAH) accounts for just five percent of the hemorrhagic strokes, but it is the deadliest of all forms of stroke with over half of all cases being fatal. 15 percent of the victims do not live long enough to reach a hospital. Another 35 percent do not survive the complications. Of those who survive, about half will have long term neurological or cognitive impairment, i.e. paralysis or stiffness, speech problems, memory loss, visual disturbances, pain, emotional difficulties, and slower thought processes. All of this boils down to me having a less than a 3.5 percent chance of writing this story.

There are two types of SAH: traumatic and spontaneous. The traumatic type is caused by an injury to the head and is not considered a stroke. The spontaneous non-traumatic SAH is commonly caused by a burst aneurysm (a sac or a bulge in a blood vessel of the brain) or the rupture of an arteriovenous malformation (or AVM, an abnormal pattern of blood vessels). This condition is thought to be present in about one in ten Americans, although a cerebral hemorrhage occurs in only about 12 percent of that population. Incidence increases with age and is probably underestimated because death is attributed to other reasons and not confirmed by autopsies. Some believe Princess Grace of Monaco died for this reason before her car crashed.

What happens in a SAH is this: blood from some pathologic process starts to collect in the fluid cavities surrounding the central nervous system, the space between the two innermost membranes covering the outer layer of brain tissue (the subarachnoid space). It is an active part of the blood-brain barrier and, normally, your nervous system is inaccessible to blood cells. This area serves as the communication channel where nerve signals and hormones travel from your brain to the rest of your body. It is not nice to have it cluttered up with blood.

Enough biology, let's move on to the part about luck. When a stroke is suspected, the goal of early assessment is to determine the cause. Treatment varies according to the underlying cause of the stroke. Ideally, people who have had a stroke of any kind are admitted to a "stroke unit," a ward in a hospital staffed by nurses and therapists with experience in stroke treatment. People admitted to a stroke unit have a higher chance of surviving than those admitted elsewhere – even to a hospital under the care of doctors without experience in stroke. The blood thinners administered to break the clots of white ischemic stroke (85 percent of all strokes) would be fatal if given to the victims of a red hemorrhagic stroke (what I had).

Homburg University Clinic is just such a place and its just 30 minutes away from the Landstuhl Army Hospital. I was very lucky that over the last 60 years such a fully integrated system of cooperation had been established between the US military community and the local German community health services. The CT scan of my head performed at Landstuhl had rapidly identified a hemorrhagic stroke by showing the blood around my brain. The results from the CT scan at Landstuhl told the doctors at Homburg what initial treatment was required.

When I got to the stroke unit, about three hours after the first symptoms had incapacitated me, time was irrelevant to me and so was the English language. I was now a patient in the intensive care stroke unit of a German teaching hospital (the University Hospital of Saarland). If I wanted something, I had to ask in German. If they wanted me to do something they said it in German. The point was fairly moot anyway at this stage because the experts were pretty much doing with me as they pleased and I didn't get to vote.

I had been in the intensive ward for no more than 30 minutes and it was time for my first angiography to confirm the diagnosis and to identify the site of the bleeding and determine what to do next. A young doctor explained the details to my wife who was at my side, who then turned to me and said, "I'll be with you. It'll be OK," and with her holding my hand, I was wheeled off to the next stop. The stroke unit surgeons were going to search for the aneurysm or the AVM and when found, seal it to prevent further bleeding.

A cerebral angiography (also known as arteriogram) is the most detailed test and the best way to diagnose the source of a hemorrhage. The test reveals the location and characteristics of the feeding arteries and draining veins. It starts with a small incision where the leg joins the hip and a thin tube is inserted into an artery in the groin. This tube is threaded up toward the brain to the major blood vessels. Dye is then injected into the blood vessels of the brain and X-rays are taken of the head, from different angles, to image the vasculature (blood vessels) of the brain. Risks of the procedure are quite low, but do include such complications as bleeding from the artery in the leg, injury to the artery in the leg, and stroke or death from the dislodging of debris within the arteries supplying the brain.

An elevator carried us down and opened onto a corridor where there was special room that reminded me of a TV studio. My wife let go of my hand. We both had to let go and assume the helpless blank stares of people on opposite sides of a closed door waiting for the unknown. There was a huge machine with a set of monitors and another bank of computers behind a wall of glass panels. As the technician was shaving the pubic hair on my right side, I was asked if I wanted to be sedated during the procedure he was about to perform. No need to play the hero now, I was able to answer, "*Ja, Gute Idee!*" About one hour after that, I found myself lying back in the hospital bed in the intensive care ward with a pressure bandage on my right leg and catheter up my dick. I don't know how long I was "out" but I remember someone telling me that they hadn't found anything. They couldn't get clear pictures of my entire brain. There was too much uncontained blood blocking their view. A second angiography would be required after the blood had time to settle – about ten days was the estimate.

Meanwhile, the day had turned to night; my wife had been there the entire time, waiting anxiously out in the corridor for word of the test results. A doctor called her into the ward and gave her the news – this night would determine what kind of statistic I would become. Now it was time for her to kiss me good-bye and go look for some way to get home. She had come in the ambulance and was now stuck in the middle of nowhere at night. Her husband had been tucked away with an uncertain future in the intensive ward. Who knows what thoughts she was thinking at that point in her long day as she waited for the taxi?

After she left, I found myself alone in the intensive ward lying on my back with wires attached to my chest. Instead of her hand, it was an armband that tightened around my right arm every few minutes as if it had a mind of its own. The pain in my head was still very intense and I remember asking the attendant if I could turn onto my side. I felt like curling up in the fetal position. He answered, "Sure, just don't go into the fetal position." Obviously, I was not his first stroke patient. A short time later, I was asleep.

This stage of my stroke was very unsettling. By this time, I knew what was happening to me, but the doctors were saying nothing more could be done for the moment. They couldn't proceed to surgery because they couldn't see where the leak was coming from. I had to lay there in the intensive stroke unit, vaguely aware that things were not settled. The goal of surgery for subarachnoid bleeding is to reduce the chances of a second bleed, which is often fatal. A common procedure, called "coiling," involves inserting coiled wires into the aneurysm. The coils are put in place using a catheter that is inserted into an artery and threaded up to the aneurysm in the brain. This procedure does not require the skull to be opened. By slowing blood flow through the aneurysm, the coil promotes clot formation, which seals off the aneurysm and prevents it from rupturing. This neuroendovascular surgery is often done at the same time as the angiography, if the aneurysm is diagnosed. Less commonly, a metal clip is placed across the aneurysm: "clipping" prevents blood from entering the aneurysm and eliminates the risk of rupture. This procedure involves opening the skull to expose the aneurysm and placing a clip to prevent more blood leaking from the affected artery.

I remained under close observation in the intensive unit for the first 24 hours with an experienced nurse checking on me each hour. Not all people suffering from hemorrhagic strokes have to undergo neurosurgery. Obviously, for some it is too late. For others, when the intracranial pressure and their overall condition do not worsen, keeping their blood pressure, blood sugar, and oxygenation at optimum levels is the normal treatment. These signs are monitored very carefully and when things appear stabilized after the first 24 hours, it is safe enough to move them out of the ISU to a monitoring unit. This is what happened to me the next afternoon.

The hours had passed quickly with me sleeping on and off most of the day. Then, in my somewhat hazy drugged condition, I heard the changeover briefing between the responsible doctors: "Absolute bed rest. He is our raw egg." I wasn't sure I liked my skull being described as a raw egg but I gladly traded in my catheter for a plastic urine bottle. I was still wearing only the military hospital gown for clothing and the standard arm band identification from the military, which brought some curious laughs from the new crew when they saw it. "We usually see those things only on babies here." I told them the Army has a way of misplacing its patients and the armband allows them to be returned to the right ward when eventually found.

My headache was still unbearable and I was receiving strong painkillers. Bed rest with no exertion is essential for stroke victims. Intravenous fluid is given to keep blood pressure at levels low enough to avoid further hemorrhage and high enough to maintain blood flow to the damaged parts of the brain. Oxygen tubes in the nostrils scare the relatives but are necessary in the early stages to make sure the brain is getting enough of the stuff. More cables attached to my chest, a blood pressure sleeve on my arm, and a clothespin-like clip grabbing my fourth finger provided round-the-clock data to the nurses' station. Analgesics such as opioids are given to control the severe headache. Stool softeners are given to prevent straining during bowel movements. A miracle drug called nimodipine (a calcium channel blocker) is taken to prevent vasospasm, the body's natural reaction to seal off blood vessels to a wound, something that would cause more brain damage in the case of SAH.

This is the condition I was in when my wife returned to the intensive unit after work the next afternoon only to find someone else lying in my bed! Imagine the thoughts that go through a loved one's head at that moment. After getting over her initial shock, she found someone who told her that I had been moved to the new room and a doctor came by to brief her again. Later that day, she called our two children to tell them what had happened in the last 24 hours. They dropped what they were doing in their own busy lives to come to the hospital the next day, nearly a 2-hour drive one way for each of them. Between the three of them, someone was with me each afternoon every day thereafter.

On the third or fourth day, as Bruce Springsteen sings "I woke up with the sheets soaking wet and a freight train running through the middle of my head," It was very warm and I was soaking the hospital linens with sweat. I told one male nurse that my headache was worse. He said, "Oh, it is nothing, stop complaining" and walked out (more on this oddball later.) Feeling the nurses were busy, I hesitated for a long time to get someone else to ask. Eventually, I reached for the call button when the pain became overpowering. The experienced nurse, thinking of possible infection, checked for fever. I had none, so she passed my concern on to a doctor in case there was a second bleed. I was still on a steady drip of dipidolor, a synthetic opioid with three fourths the potency of morphine. The doctors hesitated to give me more medication. The way my head was feeling though, I believe I could have used that other fourth as well! I was obviously showing a good deal more pain compared to the previous days.

The decision was made to run a control CT scan. My bed and I were wheeled down to the x-ray room. I slid over onto the examination table (still in my military hospital gown, exposing the family jewels to all within range, but hey, this was Europe!) and propped my head into the brace affixed to the table. The table advanced into the circular opening of the device until my head and neck were inside. The donut shaped device x-rays sections of the head in an arc as you pass through the middle of the donut. Some loud noise from the spinning components lasted about 20 minutes and then I was loaded back into the bed and returned to my room. I heard the results a short time later: The blood was more diffused than in the original scan, but there was no increase in volume. I thought to myself and to my guardian angel "thank goodness no new bleeding" – the extreme pain must have come from me, perhaps, reaching a bit too energetically for something that had fallen under the bed and shaking that cerebral fluid up so it touched some new nerve endings. Again, take it from me: at this stage, when the doctor has said "strict bed rest," it means lie flat in the bed – all the time. Ask a nurse for help if you need anything – even if you have to wait awhile for one to show up. They have had a look into your head and know what it takes to put things like blood back into the right places.

Every day during the first week a young female technician with beautiful, thick hair wheeled in a special ultrasound device called a transcranial doppler. One of the serious complications after subarachnoid hemorrhage is the occurrence of vasospasms in the basal brain arteries. This condition usually occurs between the third and fifth day after the hemorrhage. The arteries start to narrow and there is a risk of an additional, ischemic stroke as blood is prevented from getting to the brain. She could see and hear immediately in that blurry, black and white image on the monitor before her if there was any abnormal rush or narrowing going on up there behind my ears. "Scientists will save us all." The nimodipine was working and I had avoided one of the deadliest complications.

~~~~~~~~~~~~~~~

Over the next two weeks, more tests – the MRI – another coffin-like tube – another test – wide awake. Still looking for the source of my bleed. This time as he straps my head down the specialist gives me a rubber bulb to squeeze if I find I "don't like it in there" – in other words, if I panic. I was getting used to these loud tubes, I didn't panic. Although I was wearing earplugs, this machine's noise is deafening. The rhythms arrive as incessant thumps to my head. I tried counting the beats. Three long blasts of sound, followed by 6 lighter taps. I had just gotten used to this when the speed hammer started up. Just when you are getting ready to squeeze the bulb because you can't take it any longer, the noise stops and you are transported back out. I can imagine this machine is particularly scary to an elderly patient. But we all submit to the temporary discomfort because of the better accuracy in detecting changes that occur after a stroke. The MRI is less sensitive in detecting acute subarachnoid bleeding than the CT, but more sensitive in diagnosing AVM or aneurysm.

When other tests are unable to locate a source, the doctors perform a lumbar puncture, or spinal tap, to search for other possible underlying causes. A needle is inserted into the lower spine to extract a small vial full of cerebrospinal fluid or CSF. It doesn't hurt as much as you think it should - sort of like taking blood. This is the same clear fluid that surrounds your brain and flows throughout the central nervous system. It surrounds the neurons that send the signals for your legs to walk or your tongue to talk. The analysis of the fluid can also confirm hemorrhage when blood is found where normally, there should be none. After the analysis came back, there was blood in the fluid, but no bacterial or viral infections were there to be blamed for the bleeding which led to my stroke.

The second angiography was performed on the twelfth day, after the blood had sufficiently settled to allow a more complete view of the area. A doctor came to my bedside the evening before the scheduled procedure to explain the risks and have me sign the form saying I agreed to it anyway. He said that if all goes well there are two possible outcomes: we find something this time and we fix it, or we don't find anything. "Oh," I said. "Which is the preferred outcome?" Ordinarily you would hope they find it, for if they find the source they can fix it. On the other hand, as the doctor explained - if they don't find it, there is no longer anything there to fix. Well, that wasn't really reassuring to me at the time.

Early the next morning the ward received a call from radiology. A male nurse came in, grabbed the end of my bed and whisked me away to the angiography room: down the elevator into the basement, parked and left alone in the hallway to wait - for what seemed like half an hour staring at the white walls and the panels in the dropped ceiling - until the "TV" crew inside were ready for me. The bed remained in the hallway as I was transferred to a wooden palette for the test. This time, the angiography was performed by a doctor obviously well versed in torture techniques. No sedatives were even offered this time. Again, I was strapped down on the rack and inserted into the tube. He rested his hand on my hip bone for support as he fed the catheter through my arteries. Somehow this human contact and his steady nerves comforted me as I was immobilized in that alien environment. He proceeded to push his tools up through my vessels to reach his intended target, but he needed to coordinate with the technicians behind the panels taking the pictures. I could see and hear them smoking and joking with someone who just popped in for a chat. At least that is what I was thinking as the patient. Meanwhile, I had some wire running from my groin up into my skull and it seemed the doctor had to interrupt their small talk at the right moment to get them ready to film the next injection. I asked myself, "How can someone just walk in at a time like this? What aren't they paying attention? Isn't this the only game in town? Why does he (we) have to wait?" I had been told not to move my head and tried not to think about anything.

The doctor was very calm and it all worked out fine. There were six injections. I could feel every squirt of the iodine dye as he injected it into the blood vessels of my brain. I am sure this procedure has to produce an increase pressure in the brain – *'cause it hurt like hell!* It felt warm if not even hot, but it lasted only a short time and I was used to head pain by then anyway. They were obviously looking at the areas behind my eyes, then behind my cheekbones and ears, then my jaw and the back of my tongue. First came three shots in sequence up the right side then three more down the left side. I don't know this for sure. But that is what I felt and boy, was I glad when it was over. I have never blacked out or tried hallucinogenic drugs, but I saw what it must be like during this procedure. With my eyes closed, it was as if the channel suddenly changed and I saw a steady pattern of pure, bright white lines against a pitch black background – a black and white rhombic pattern like the outlines of cell boundaries. Is this what a 10 on the scale of pain looks like?

Back in my room on the ward, the doctor told me they still didn't find the source of the blood. He explained my case as one of "self -healing." No amount of testing could find an explanation for the source of the blood in my brain. There was nothing to coil, nothing to clip. I liked the way this story was developing.

Now the testing designed to assess any nerve and reflex damage began. I was wheeled to various examination rooms and hooked up from head to toe as they applied little suction cups that send electrical currents out. They passed a magnetic wand over my head that emitted a pulse to time the speed of the signals to and from the brain. In one test, I was supposed to be completely relaxed. Just as I would start to relax, a phone would ring, her colleague would crash in to ask how much longer it would take, or the jack hammer of the construction crew in the hallway would blast away. "Try to relax," said the technician not looking up from her monitoring screen as if immune to these distractions. "Oh, sure thing" I said shaking my head in disbelief.

According to the doctors, my headache would last another 4-6 weeks. They were still giving me the nimodipine pills and the daily wake-up calls, which consisted of a familiar tapping on my hand every morning (at 5:00 a.m.!) as an understanding face appeared at my bedside, holding a needle in their hand and looking for a vein or artery to take another blood sample. Eventually, they ran out of tests to perform, but I was relieved when they decided to keep me at the stroke unit for a while longer.

"In the sick room, ten cents' worth
of human understanding equals ten
dollars' worth of medical science."

Martin H. Fischer

G. M. PEACH

CHAPTER 4

Between tests

The Germans say *"Schlaf dich gesund,"* which translates to "Sleep yourself back to health." During the initial days and weeks in the stroke unit, I just wanted people to let me sleep. The need to sleep is one of the big things that a stroke does to you, so that is pretty much all I did between meals. Doing anything else seemed to hurt. When asleep, the brain has time to make some sense of the stimulation it's received: it can try to organize and file information and begin the calm healing process it requires. Lying there in the bed, all of my senses seemed to be on some maximum setting. Sounds were too loud and chaotic. Touch was too sensitive. Light was too bright. Nevertheless, I thought things were going well – until a new roommate was wheeled in for observation on the second night.

He was a young soccer player who had headed a ball and then passed out on the field. He had visitors from the moment he entered my room, and they all wanted to relive the play of the game and celebrate his regaining consciousness by all talking at once. Every sound seemed twice as loud in my head. It was almost tolerable as long as my morphine drip was working. It didn't seem to bother the nurse on duty. She let it go on even after I complained. Of course, when I told my Teutonic wife about this the next day, she wanted to go looking for that nurse and dress her up and down drill sergeant style for being so insensitive and not taking care of me, but I was able to talk her out of it with my reasoning that you catch more flies with honey than with vinegar and, I didn't want to begin what was to be a long in-patient stay with a fight. Fortunately, another room became available the next day and he was moved. The soccer team could party elsewhere.

The doctor visited once a day to share my test results and check on my progress. I fell easily into the daily rhythms of the nursing staff and actually looked forward to the regular meals of bland hospital food. I adjusted to sleeping with the colored cables with suction cup endings and a pressure sleeve constantly monitoring my blood pressure. I learned what the various lines on the oscilloscope represented: blue for oxygen level, yellow for frequency of respiration, green for pulse rate. I could watch the level of the fluid in the IV bottles dropping as the hours went by. I was not allowed, nor did I even want, to sit up alone or leave the bed. The door to the hallway was usually left open during the daytime. In case there was a change in the vital signs, nurses would be better able to hear the alarm signal. My own ears delivered the sounds of the "outside world" - the occasional calls and wails of other patients and the beeping of other monitors in other rooms. I knew which beeps would bring a nurse running and which were not so critical. I knew what time the shift change was and when the nurses took their break. I could hear the elevator that delivered the meal trays, and knew that in a short while I would be eating more bread, diet cheese, and yoghurt.

All of this was new and, sometimes, embarrassing for me. I had never spent a day on any hospital ward before this happened. The nurses do it every day, for up to 30 patients – most of whom are older and in worse shape than I was. In spite of all that, they were usually friendly and generally kind. At first though, I found myself getting irritated when someone came to check on my neighbor or to record the readings from the monitors, without seeing my needs, i.e., that my water jug was empty, my urine jug was full, the window shade was open with the sun beating directly into my eyes, or my pillow needed a good fluffing after a sweaty afternoon. From my initial experience in the intensive care unit with the hourly visits, I thought their routines would include frequent stops at my bedside to take care of such things. How dependent we are on the assistance of total strangers for nearly everything! And, how we appreciate the motivation and quality of some hospital personnel in the way they approach each task – and learn to accept the lack of it in others.

Now, when I look back on this period, I see things a little differently. Perhaps the cause of my irritation at the time was not that they were "ignoring" my comfort. Maybe I was just not aware that my brain perceived these as interruptions, unexpected and unproductive intrusions into my own "self-healing" time. Perhaps I needed my solitude more than a pillow fluffing after all. This is when I was using the pain in my head as a mental challenge. I was trying to ignore it or minimize it by concentrating on it. I was willing it out of the fluid spaces where it did not belong. I was alone and trying to do this when the door would open and someone would come in to do something for my neighbor and leave. The staff was not being insensitive; it just wasn't on their plan to visit me.

Between feedings and washings, the rest of these days were for me, alone with myself, lying on my back trying to re-calibrate. I think I was meditating, to block out external influences so that my mind could focus on my brain, where the problem was. I didn't have to think about yesterday or tomorrow. I just had to repair the spot that had broken and flush the blood out of those places it didn't belong. Just as I had done in my car outside the classroom, I was asking my mind to take charge of a real mess up there in my brain. I was really breaking my days into time slots for "events" and "non-events." The events included the three meal times, the morning hygiene, and the physical therapy. The non-events were even more important for me. I was stretching time into the longest possible interval before popping a pain killer. I was trying to sleep it out while building strength for the next event. As my wife later told me, I was not much fun to be with that first week.

It took me a few days to realize that it is perfectly OK to push the call button to the nurses' station for some needed assistance. Once I discovered this, I never had to wait long for someone to come. They were in the other rooms doing the same things I wanted them to do in my room. I was also struggling with the subject of how to go about answering nature's call for the big one. For the life of me I couldn't picture how it would be possible to accomplish from my prostrate position. On the fourth or fifth day, it was literally time as they say, "to shit or get off the pot." I worked up the courage to ask the male nurse who had seemed most understanding up to that point. He said, "Haven't you made a bowel movement yet?" After no great discussion, he left and returned shortly with a large, COLD, stainless steel pot, which he shoved under the sheet to the proper position and left me alone. A few minutes later, I was pushing the call button again for I really needed some assistance, if you know what I mean. Without a lot of talk or action, he took care of the most natural thing in the world, cleaned me up and left. Out in the hall, I heard someone joke about chocolate pudding. I was glad that everything came out alright (pun intended) and once again impressed by the staff's focus on the patient and respect for the dignity of the individual.

One of my first memories of those early days was of the man opposite me in the room after the soccer player left. He was 63 and couldn't pronounce a single word clearly. He was also unable to walk. There was always a curtain separating us so I never did see him. I listened as the nurses talked with him and tried to understand his sounds when they brought his food or washed him. I knew his name was Mr. Schneider. That is the most common name in Germany, like Smith is for us. I listened through the curtain one day as his son sat beside him and tried to activate his Dad's mobile phone so he could receive and send text messages. The man could not utter the pin number requested by the son. The young man tried the same question again and again, but got the same response - nothing. He had such patience and there were such long moments of silence, as father and son sat together in thought. It almost made me cry. Two men were sitting together – one not knowing what to say, the other unable to say it.

After a week, I was moved to a room a few doors further away from the intensive ward. Nurses encouraged me to perform self-care tasks such as eating and shaving, as early as medically possible. One day a friendly nurse told me to carefully get out of the bed and sit on the chair she had just placed next to the bed, so she could change the linen. Up until then, I had been rolling over on one side as she pushed the clean sheets under me, and then rolling back onto the now clean side while she finished the second half. As the days went on, we synchronized our schedules so that I would be out and about at the time they were changing the bed. I think the personnel are sincerely happy to see one of their patients making strides to recovery.

I still had a good amount of stiffness in my left leg and neck. But, freed of my cables, I was well enough to explore the stroke unit on my own and make my way from my new room to the corridor toilette. Sometimes I felt the little jab in the throat when swallowing and thought how easily we all take for granted the act of swallowing. My headache had settled into a predictable and tolerable pattern of its own. If I was not sleeping, rather than just staring blankly out the window, I would pass the rest of my time focusing on the print of a paperback, another form of meditation to tune out the pain. Concentration and focus was still a problem. I was only able to read a few sentences at a time before putting the book down. It was a mystery novel and I nodded off, imagining where the lost treasure that the main characters were looking for might be hidden.

I had the new room to myself for a day or two before another roommate showed up. He was 10 years older than me, apparently in good physical shape, and also being treated for stroke. He too got away without an operation, but seemed to have some slight trouble speaking and walking. He had been a welder all his life at a nearby global equipment manufacturer and smoked a couple packs a day. He showed me an unopened pack of Marlboros which he said, with a little pride and a little disbelief, had remained that way – unopened – all week. He kept them in his shirt pocket, probably a habit of his for the last 40 years, as a test of his willpower. He told me how much his left leg had improved and asked me to join him for his daily exercise routine walking the two flights of stairs to the lobby and back. He had to work on keeping the "numb" foot from landing in front of the good foot and tripping himself. My own steps had to be very deliberate as I followed him down the stairs and held on to the railing. I took him as a sort of role model for recovery and found it a good way to pass some time.

Summer arrived in Germany at about the same time as my stroke. The weather changed overnight from rainy, cold, and grey to warm, sunny, and blue. The first week I was in the hospital, the temperature rose from 50 to 85 degrees with crystal blue skies visible through the windows. Or maybe the warmth and hopeful skies were brought to me by my wife. She is a very generous, kind, and caring person. Every day after she got off work, my wife made the 45 minute drive to the hospital. She brought me some clean, loose fitting clothes and put a flower from our backyard garden in a glass jar on the windowsill. It added some color to the room and made me realize how time and nature were going on without me. It reminded me that life was happening outside. I had not even thought about it and it surprised me to realize I had been "away" from my life for so long. I really had not missed a thing: no phones ringing, no TV, no work deadline approaching. My brain was busy repairing itself and I was letting it do its thing. The strawberries had now ripened in the fields and on another visit, my wife and I shared a bowl full together. It was a real tasty treat and a welcome change from the standard hospital food. When I awoke and saw the flower and the blue skies outside, I thought how lucky I was. I had survived a brain bleed and I have a wife and two children standing by me through this, reassuring me, taking care of me, and urging me to get well.

This was a totally new experience for us all. No one prepares loved ones for such an emotional event and expectations may vary considerably. I never thought about it from her perspective. She could not imagine it from my perspective. It is only natural that after the initial scare when the doctors told her what was wrong that my wife should be looking for her own peace. With the word "stroke," life is broken apart. She wanted to know if there was anything she could do. She wanted to talk. She wanted to know what type of survivor would be coming home to live with her.

My wife wanted me to talk, but I couldn't process any complicated emotions, even though to all outward appearances my brain seemed to be working fine. I couldn't focus for more than a few minutes without getting fatigued. My daughter tried to read to me. It hurt me to have to tell her to stop, but it was too much – the headache was too intense. I couldn't concentrate. I couldn't keep up the front. I had to sleep. I needed to be alone. They tried to touch my head in a loving, tender way, but I made them stop. It hurt. I could feel every root of my hair (what little I still have there on top). Moving into any other position caused pain in my head. Those early days were the worst period of the whole experience for all of us.

It was too early for me to exchange feelings that form in the part of the brain effected by the stroke, but my wife couldn't have known that. Her visiting hours did not coincide with my best "availability" time. She had to work all day and then drive almost 2 hours round trip to visit me. I wished she could have been there when I was feeling "up" early in the day, after the pain killers were at their peak effectiveness and before the effect wore off. Instead, she usually caught me in my irritable moods when it was near the time for the next scheduled pain killer or when the drowsiness of fatigue was setting in. My routine was actually forced upon me by the pain medication and nursing schedule and there was simply not much return on investment for my wife. Deep down I wanted her to be there, but I was powerless. Our communication suffered. She got the feeling that I didn't want her there, which was wrong. My brain just wasn't up to responding in a normal way. I just wanted or needed to feel her presence, like at the emergency room.

It pained me for my family to see me this way. Knowing they had other responsibilities, I felt guilty about making them drive so long just to hold my hand and watch me sleep, but I just didn't feel fit enough for longer visits. It was too strenuous for me at that point. Their first reaction was always to protect me and to ensure I was receiving top care from what is assumed by definition to be an under-motivated hospital staff that could never be good enough in their eyes. I looked forward to the visits from my loved ones and they were very important to me, but I needed all my strength to get control over my pain. All the action and bustling about was a distraction which seemed to increase my pain. The best thing a loved one can provide to the patient at this stage is simply a calming presence and the encouraging knowledge that someone cares and believes with the patient that patience will pay off in the long run.

Of course, friends and relatives wanted to phone or visit me after they heard what had happened to me. Family and friends have to try to understand that a stroke patient is experiencing a lot of confusion and anxiety, not to mention constant pain. My wife instinctively knew how I felt and threw up a protective screen around me. There was no need to discuss this with her for long. We agreed. I even said it would be better for me if she and my two adult kids came to visit on separate days rather than as a group. I felt bad about my "antisocial" behavior, but she could see how I was still in pain and simply not fit enough for any entertainment. I would tire easily and my concentration lasted only for short periods of about 30-40 minutes now, then I would need to fall asleep. I apologize if any feelings were hurt and hope they all understand now.

Loved ones and visitors have to remember to let the patient rest when needed. Therapy can be exhausting and they should respect the healing power of sleep for the brain. Try to accept the patient's condition at this stage and convey understanding and support for their recovery. One of the symptoms of stroke is the patient may feel smothered by well-meaning loved ones who rush to take care of everything, instead of letting patients learn how far they can progress on their own. Someone has said that "Stroke recovery is not a sprint, it is a marathon." Some stroke patients are easily frustrated and some have trouble dealing with extraneous noise or a rush of activity. Visitors should not take it personally if the patient does not respond as expected in the early stages. Remember, the patient has survived an emotional event. Step by step, day by day, they are (or should be) trying to re-wire the damaged areas of their brains. However, if the patient seems depressed, it should be discussed with the nurses. The trauma, although a physical one, can take on a more mental aspect over time.

Short tempers and more irritable moods are changes that commonly surface at some point in the stroke victims' recovery. Mine occurred during the days of the extreme pain when I had an issue with a male nurse. Funny thing now is that I cannot remember his name. I remember all the others, just not his. He had a manner that was different from the other nurses and I thought I could even see the "attitude chip" on his shoulder. It irritated me that he acted like he knew more than the doctors and assumed decisions that were above his pay grade. He hadn't even passed on my complaint of the new resurging pain to a supervisor during that week of the heat spell. Now, I could hear the voice of an elderly woman screaming or, I guess a better word is wailing, from some distance down the hallway. Between her screams came the words "Help me. Why don't you help me?"

After the screaming had gone on long enough to cause some concern among everyone within hearing distance, her words started getting louder; she was approaching out in the hallway, coming in my direction. I saw this particular male nurse and another colleague rushing by my doorway as they went to escort her back to her room. But the screaming did not stop, in fact, it sounded like a scuffle and I knew things had gotten physical. Through the split second field of vision allowed by my door frame one of the nurses returned. "Attitude man" was left to handle the situation by himself now. The screaming continued and between screams came the words, "Stop. What are you doing to me? Why are you doing this to me?" More screaming. Eventually, peace returned to the ward and "attitude man" passed by my doorway looking like an emotional wreck. Hours later I asked a nurse what had happened and how was the old lady doing now. She just said, "The heat is hard on people." I never saw attitude man again after that day.

In talking with my son as I was writing this book, I was reminded of one of my not so finest moments. It also involved attitude man – a few days before the scene with the old lady. The nurses carefully supervise the administration of the strong pain killer to ensure patients do not develop a dependency. Perhaps I am being unfair, but he really upset me one evening when he removed the dipi-drip before the bottle was empty. He threw away enough to fill at least 5 or 6 injection vials! I said, "Hey, what are you doing? That's not empty!" He said, "Yes it is," and dropped it in the trash can and walked out of the room. I was convinced he would be waiting to go through the trash when it was emptied at the end of his shift – picking out all those unemptied bottles in order to black market the stuff at the expense of patients who really needed it!

I told my son about it when he visited me later that day and insisted he get the bottle out of the trash to keep as evidence. I got a look somewhere between confusion and disbelief from my son. He didn't know just quite how to tell me he thought I was nuts. Then he told me I was being a bit unreasonable and I should try to rest. I have since learned that morphine or "Miss Emma" really does have a street value of about a dollar per milligram! Hey, with an imagination like this and some luck, I could be writing a bestselling crime novel.

In all fairness, we all give too much thought to the irritants in life. Why do the problem students always get more attention than the ones who are really trying to excel? Why do we remember the negative things first? To fix that right now let me relate a more positive memory. It involves an extraordinary member of the stroke unit staff. During the first days of my bed rest, a little pixie of a woman about 33 years old came to the room dressed in green hospital scrubs – the physical therapist. Again, I was lucky that she was there and not some other, less patient-focused therapist. She is the kind of care giver that should have the most written about them. When she finished working with my roommate who had already been there for some days, she introduced herself to me. She had a natural empathy and her enthusiasm was contagious. We hit it off right away as I am sure she also did with all her patients. I told her about the headache pain and, in particular, the pain in my lower back and left leg. She nodded as if she had been expecting that and proceeded to guide me through some exercises that didn't require me to get out of the bed and then she left. She was highly qualified and spread good cheer even when sadness would seem like the more appropriate reaction given the fate of her patients.

She came every morning after that and spread a brightness throughout the room and made me do stretches designed to keep my back and legs from getting too stiff. She saw and did what the other staff should have seen and done when they came into the room. I mean just the basics like refilling the empty water pitcher and seeing the sun shades, putting them up if it was too dark and down if the sun was in my eyes. One day I heard her come in, but I was feeling a bit depressed and hoped she would just go away. I didn't want to move. The risk of falling into depression is rather common at this point in a survivor's recovery. She wasn't about to give me a choice so after a while, I decided to sit up – for her. She just waited patiently until I took my head out of the pillow to begin the exercises. These therapists know better than us patients at that point what we are capable of doing for ourselves. I was very unsure of myself at that point. Her touch told me that I wasn't isolated and there was hope. She quickly showed me that I didn't have to adopt that sedated shuffle of the other patients, their limbs as stiff and wooden as marionettes. It was very important to me. After a few sessions, I was walking alone and learning to do the thera-band exercises out in the hallway.

The saying "as the spirit moves you" seems very appropriate here. She was showing my mind that my legs were not injured. They could move normally if my brain would only find the right connections so the signals could travel down to my leg and make the muscles move. Together, we were reprogramming my brain – giving it a positive vision of reconnecting the damaged or interrupted nerve endings. All my spirit needed to get me moving again was her guiding touch and her warm-hearted way. Up until this point, my treatment was pretty much the standard school medicine - very formal visits by a very formal doctor and nurses performing routine duties with machines and drugs providing all the answers. There was never any direct mention of alternative healing methods or neuroplasticity (more about this in the next chapter), although throughout the ordeal I felt my mind trying to will its way through to my damaged brain. The sessions with the physical therapist were essentially adjusting this mind-body relationship. I give credit to her and this treatment for the quick return of my mobility. That is what the rehabilitation phase is all about.

The stereotype of healthcare calls for a neglectful, brusque, underpaid, and indifferent staff. That may be what many patients perceive during their experience in a hospital. Everyone knows a good doctor or nurse can make a world of difference. My perception of the staff is an appreciative one. I can only hope that all stroke victims will be lucky enough to receive the kind of care and encouragement that I did.

My period of learning German medical terms and how to say "This plain yogurt is great" three times per day in German did not end when the time came for me to leave the clinic. I had watched the welder pack up his few belongings by emptying the drawers of the metal bedside table and the clothes locker into his small duffle bag – a day in advance of his discharge. Now I did the same with my stuff and waited impatiently for my wife to come collect me. We walked slowly together down the hallway to say goodbye to the professional team at the stroke unit: We left a thank you package for the nurses on duty that morning, and then left through the same door I had been stretchered through three weeks earlier.

I was on my way to a rehab center, deep in the backwoods of the German countryside. It was time to start learning more about myself and others.

"In solitude, you will find strength -
in silence, recovery."

(*"In der Einsamkeit liegt Kraft, in der
Stille Erholung."*)

German proverb

G. M. PEACH

CHAPTER 5

Recovery and rehabilitation

I don't know if these are the words of St. Wendelin, but they pretty much sum up the philosophy of the rehab center, located in the small town that bears his name. Located deep in the countryside, today St. Wendel has about 25,000 inhabitants. The town has been there since the sixth century when St. Wendelin, the son of Scottish king, settled there as a hermit on his way back from a pilgrimage to Rome. The locals credited him with saving them (and their cattle) from a few deadly plagues and eventually built a chapel over his grave where they could worship him. Today, the center is situated on the slope of a hillside overlooking rural meadows and bordering a cool forest criss-crossed by a network of walking trails. This would be my home for the next four weeks.

My wife followed the winding roads through the green countryside for just under an hour in order to drop me off for the next phase of my recovery – the Mediclin rehab center. At the reception desk I got a room assignment on the second floor and a key to my mailbox. We were sent up to the nurses' station on the second floor where a nurse gave me the pills prescribed by the Homburg doctor – one to control the blood pressure and one to lower the cholesterol and of course one really strong pain reliever for the headaches which I now took only twice per day. The nurse on duty told me I had an appointment the next morning with the head of the neurological unit. My wife had already done some research about the place, and upon hearing the name, she knew the appointment would be with the founder of the center, which is nearly 30 years old now. We found my room and I was grateful when she arranged the few clothes she had packed for me (no more sexy hospital gowns!) neatly in the wall unit. We did a quick orientation tour of the center together and then said goodbye at the main entrance. She would be back to visit on the weekend.

Sometimes it's truly best for someone recovering from stroke to do so in a rehab facility designed for that situation rather than returning straight home. One of the best ways for the family to help a loved one is to ensure the stroke patient receives rehab therapy. Incredibly, or luckily for me, my wife knew this and even while I was still in the stroke unit, she was making the phone calls and visiting the insurance provider to make sure all the paperwork was in place to ensure a smooth admission for me as an in-patient at this rehab facility. Now I was alone – by myself, but not quite myself – assigned to a private room (only single rooms are available), not knowing what a rehab center was, but in agreement that I needed one.

My first lesson presented itself a short time later that evening in the dining room. Seated alone at a table, I ate the evening meal by myself and had the opportunity to check out the other "guests." It was easy to identify the newcomers. We were the ones who were sitting alone. It was cafeteria style with hot water dispensers for tea (coffee at breakfast only), a dietary-correct main course and a salad bar, which I learned always included carrot salad if nothing else. It was very much like the large dining room of any vacation hotel except it was divided into two sections.

I quickly learned that one section was reserved with name cards for the people who needed to have their food trays brought to the table and also, in some cases, to have assistance in feeding themselves. Many of them came to the meals in wheelchairs or with walkers. On the other side, where I sat, some of the people had fresh scars stretching across the top or side of their scalp where hair had been only a few weeks earlier. I also was surprised to see so many younger and apparently fit people as well. They tended to move at full speed, talk a bit louder, and laugh when one of them told a joke. Later on, after I talked with some of them, I would learn that a nice suntan on the outside doesn't necessarily mean the sun is shining on the inside.

The next morning I was called in to the doctor's office for the entrance examination nearly on time. The doctor is in his mid-60's, short with a full, angular trimmed beard like Gregory Peck had as Cap'n Ahab in the film *Moby Dick*. He is forthright and friendly and, after browsing through my file, offers to speak English with me. I respond that this is a good idea and before starting his examination, he briefly explained the hemorrhage is sometimes caused by a small defect or lesion that is not detected because it has already sealed itself off. The exact mechanism and why it leaves no trace are unknown. Then he begins the examination. I am told to walk back and forth across the room for him. He notices something not quite right in the way I position my left foot. I touch my nose with my index fingers and follow his index finger with my eyes as he studies their movement. He strokes my palms and the bottom of my feet with a cold, sharp pointed instrument. I feel it all. Good sign. The reflexes in both ankles, however, are not there and he thought my right eye (or was it the left one?) seemed to straggle along out of step behind his finger. And, that is that, the test is over.

This all indicates the location of damage was deep within the brain where important motor and sensory signal neurons are relayed to control hearing, sight, eye movement and body movement as well as blood pressure and emotions.

Well, I can see and I can walk and the mini Gregory Peck tells me I must learn to enjoy my leisure time. "How very perceptive on his part," I thought to myself: "How did he know that I had no real hobbies and that I used my free time to look for new clients or new software to improve my business?" Little did I know at that moment he was actually referring to the fairly sparse, daily schedule he envisioned for me over the next four weeks! In fact, for the remainder of that first week, my daily calendar was nearly blank.

Stroke rehabilitation actually starts as soon as possible in the hospital. When patients are stable, as I was, rehabilitation may begin within two days after the stroke has occurred. I was fortunate that the Homburg clinic had already started my "pre-rehab" with such a capable physical therapist. Now I would have the chance to continue this therapy over the next few weeks and experience healing along with my fellow patients. It was an eye-opener for me to learn that not everyone was there to recover from stroke. Some were being treated for brain injuries, white stroke, MS, tinnitus, and PTSD. Of course, a few of them were "old hands" returning to the rehab center for treatments again after having been there in prior years for the same illnesses. One young girl in her twenties had been diagnosed with MS - incurable. No one seemed to talk about their individual illnesses at first, which I suppose is the least stressful approach. Nevertheless, each of them had a reason for being at the rehab center: stroke, brain trauma or tumor operation,

MS, tinnitus, burn out syndrome, etc. It was a strange and novel feeling for me to think of so many seemingly average people affected by crippling illness being in one place – each with their own fears and challenges.

There's still so much we don't know about how the brain compensates for the damage caused by stroke or brain attack. It is possible that some individual areas of the brain are destroyed while others continue to function. It may be that the ability to speak or to feel or to think coherently is shut down, while other areas responsible for certain motoric functions, like walking or using the hands, can be reactivated. Decades of scientific research now show that rehabilitation is critical for optimal stroke recovery. It always depends on the extent of the brain damage and the scope of the therapeutic treatments.

Mainstream medicine is unable to understand or explain more than just a few of the mind-body relationships at work in each unique human being. Scientists have only recently discovered that the human brain can change itself. Development does not stop after childhood. The idea that the brain can change its own structure through thought and activity is a fairly new model known today as neuroplasticity. Neuro is for "neuron," the nerve cells in our brains that create impulses for all kinds of mental functions – muscle control, sensory perception memory, emotions, and speech – which are sent out through the nervous system. Plastic is for "changeable, malleable, modifiable."

There are examples of people who have had strokes and been declared incurable, who were helped many years later to recover with neuroplastic treatments. The damage is not irreversible as previously thought. The benefits come from helping the brain to reorganize itself with physical therapy in peaceful surroundings, which in turn helps the stroke survivor (or the tinnitus patient, etc.) to recover lost brain functions. I believe I was instinctively practicing neuroplastic techniques in my surroundings from day one.

Damage control is the art of taking a difficult matter and making sure that it does not get worse. Some brain cells may be only temporarily damaged, not killed, and may resume functioning. In some cases, the brain can reorganize its own functioning. Sometimes, a region of the brain "takes over" for a region damaged by the stroke. Some stroke survivors experience remarkable and unanticipated recoveries that can't be explained. At any rate, this seemed like the right place to practice damage control and it seemed my rehabilitation program was going to be focused on ensuring that I do nothing to make things worse in this phase of recovery. I was about to start revising my understanding of leisure time.

The patients go to the lobby every morning to check their mailbox for any eventual changes in their daily activities schedule. As I said, mine was nearly empty for the first few days. Over the weekend, I browsed through a pamphlet offered at the front desk that listed all the different therapies available at the center along with a few motivational quotes like "Laziness is the habit of taking your break before you get tired." The handout consisted of ten full pages and was organized alphabetically from A to Z. It included everything from audio coping to pension advice. I focused immediately on the letter C and the words "Classic Massage" and asked where to sign up. "It is not a wish list, sir," I was politely informed. "The doctor has to approve each treatment or therapy session as part of your integrated plan." "Oh, what a shame," I said to myself. (I never did get on the list for a massage.)

When I got my first weekly schedule, I was relieved to find the doctor had taken away some of my leisure time and filled it with measured doses of exercise. Performing any strenuous weight training was forbidden, leaving mostly mobility and relaxation activities on the program. I was not too pleased when I saw the first activity was scheduled to start at 7:00 a.m. (the breakfast meal didn't even start until 8:00)! Even back in the stroke unit we got a cup of coffee (with the breakfast yogurt) before anything else happened in the morning.

It would be boring for most readers if I were to describe here the daily routine and events at the rehab center in detail. Gee whiz, it was pretty boring for me while I was living it! But then again, that is just what I needed in order to continue my recovery. The activities described below are just a small sampling of the therapies the center offers depending on what illness is being treated:

Back and stretching exercises. You all know the advice: Exercising just 30 minutes per day can do wonders for your health. It has been shown to lower the risk of heart attack and stroke. A program of regular exercise can help lower blood pressure and reduce cholesterol build-up in the blood vessels (arteriosclerosis). My schedule said 7:00 a.m. - mat exercises. I had to wake up and go down stairs to join the group on the floor mats or sit on one of the exercise balls as the instructor talked a small group of us through a series of stretching and loosening up exercises. It is a great way to wake up before enjoying that first cup of coffee, and I still enjoy this routine at home (well, OK, not at 7:00 a.m.)

Water exercises. The center had a fairly large, indoor swimming pool. A diverse group of about 25-30 people were scheduled at the same time for water gymnastics to perform range of motion exercises. The idea here is to exercise safely while placing less stress on the joints as your weight is partially supported by the water. It was pretty funny to see adults, ranging in age from 45 to 70, splashing about and laughing like children as they "bicycled" a spray of water into the air while hanging on to the side of the pool, or hopped across the width of the pool by high-knee lunges.

Physical therapy. I am always intrigued at how these experienced specialists can always find the exact point on your body that is giving you the problem with their first grip. "Ouch," I said, as she pushed down on my first rib after listening to me complain of the continuing stiffness on the left side of my neck. She started right there under my collarbone and then worked her way up each of the muscle groups leading into the base of the skull. They can usually guess what kind of a job you have just from watching how you sit or how you shake hands. In my case, it was the "turtle neck" of someone who works at a computer all day and doesn't exercise to balance the strain on those particular muscles. Again, they taught me some good exercises which I continue to perform now at home.

Cycle ergometer. This activity is another good choice for people trying to manage their high blood pressure. A few times per week I had to go to a small room that contained six stationary bicycles. There was a steady flow of patients coming and going, but I never had to wait for a bike. An exercise bike (essentially a bike without wheels) is a low impact, safe way to study the effect of exercise on the cardio-vascular system. A therapist measures blood pressure before and after cycling at about 25 kmh for a period of twenty minutes and that's it. My first few times doing this showed that the blood pressure pills I was taking were not nearly effective enough, both systolic and diastolic shot up to hypertension levels. The doctor changed the dosage of my medication and then I had no problem riding the bike. This was great news as I had plans for the future to take a 10-day bike tour with some friends. I would have to get my time per day up quite a bit from 20 minutes before then, but I felt good.

Relaxation therapy. This is incredible! I cannot rave enough about this discovery. I learned something about stress and how it can affect your health even when all the while you are not even aware that you have stress. Stress management, including mind-body relaxation techniques, appears to be useful in lowering the risk of future stroke. Increased stress and the accompanying decrease in relaxation time, leads to higher levels of stress hormones within your body - hormones such as adrenaline and cortisol that shut down other functions. Your brain behaves differently, affecting the memory and your body's self-healing abilities. Stress hormones are linked indirectly to stroke risk. A one-time stressful event rarely causes a stroke, but long-term unresolved stress can contribute to high blood pressure. Relaxation techniques include behavioral therapeutic approaches that differ widely in philosophy, methodology, and practice. All acknowledge the effects that the mind can have on the body. Research suggests that relaxation therapy may even help stroke victims recover more rapidly. I certainly support that premise!

My sessions at the rehab center were conducted in groups of 6-10 people and lasted about 50 minutes. The primary goal is the adoption of a passive attitude towards intruding thoughts and a return to the focus, usually a repetitive focus (on a word, sound, prayer phrase, or muscular activity). The focus we used was our own body, lying flat on our backs on foam exercise mats. In a calm and soothing voice, the instructor started us on a journey examining the surface sensations and the insides of our entire body. Our concentration was directed first at our toes then on to the heel, ankle, shin, knee and so on, proceeding upwards, very slowly, visualizing each major segment all the way up the spine to the face, eye sockets, and scalp. There was one fellow who just couldn't stand the quiet: He stood up, grabbed his shoes, and said he had to go to the men's room. He never did come back to that class. Don't be like him. Do some form of relaxation therapy once a day for 15-20 minutes and you will soon notice how much better you feel and how much more capable you are when you finish.

Speech therapy. You have to remember, I was performing all these therapy sessions with the instructors speaking German. So when it came time for my appointment with the speech therapist, I just couldn't resist having a little fun with her. Cap'n Ahab arranged the appointment for me as a result of my entrance exam when it seemed I was having a little trouble mixing the letters b, r, and v in words as I spoke, i.e., "I'm veby sovy to disturv you." Speech therapists can help people who develop aphasia after a brain attack that does not cause progressive damage. Aphasia is the partial or complete loss of the ability to express or understand spoken or written language. It results from damage to the areas of the brain that control language, but the nature and degree of the difficulty vary, which reflects the complex nature of our language function. So anyway, when the therapist introduced herself to me and asked what my problem was, I declared in my very best German that ever since my stroke I had an inexplicable American accent and asked if she could eliminate that and restore me to an accent-free German. As everyone knows, the Germans have no sense of humor so I suppose it is not entirely a credit to my German that she did not take it as a joke. She was seriously considering how to begin treatment when I laughed and said I was just kidding and admitted to my American roots. She quickly informed me that, in fact, such cases of waking up with previously unrecognized language features are a well-documented occurrence after stroke. I didn't know that it even has a name, the "foreign accent syndrome." Well, in that session, which took place four weeks after the stroke, I must not have needed any words that contained the letters b, r, or v. We agreed that my speech was no longer affected and no further sessions to treat aphasia were necessary. She even said she liked my American accent!

At this stage of my recovery, it sometimes felt like I had a thin, transparent veil around my head. It now seemed like my senses of hearing and vision were being muffled or softened by some invisible filter, like the stimuli were bouncing off a few extra places before being processed by my brain. I couldn't hear direction. I may have looked behind and to the left when the source was actually somewhere to my front right. Even when outside on a beautiful sunny day, light was never bright, but always somehow matted as if viewed through a veil. It wasn't bad and not dangerous, but it often made me strangely uncomfortable after the super sensitivity I had experienced at the beginning.

Overall, the atmosphere at the rehab clinic was nice. It was designed to be stress-free and it was. I had no TV in my room, but a TV room was set up for the World Cup Soccer Championship and I was able to watch a few of the matches there. I went down to watch the Netherlands play Brazil. With the absence of the US Team, someone got the idea that I must be from Holland because of my obvious non-German accent. From then on I was the "Dutchman" everywhere I went. They knew it wasn't true, but it was well-intentioned and broke the ice and brought us all a bit closer. Mobile phones were only allowed in the private rooms or outside the building. It was truly relaxing to be able to walk around so many people without seeing or hearing anyone using a cell phone. Think about it: no one talking into thin air, no stupid customized ringtones vibrating through the room, people not staring at their hands but actually looking at what's happening socially around them. In my room, I remembered my pin and even got to be pretty good at the texting function, which, I admit, I had never tried to use before. Now, I used it to be "closer" with loved ones living their busy lives far away.

Shortly after I entered the rehab clinic, I received a text message from my son. He signed "Dad" and I knew I was a grandfather. He told me the baby was a healthy little girl. At the start of my illness, his wife had been in the ninth month of her pregnancy. She had cheered me up and given me real motivation to recover quickly when she told me she would hold out giving birth until I was out of danger and out of the hospital. She is a woman of her word! I was barely out of the hospital with my condition improving when my granddaughter was born – about 4 days late – a healthy, 8-lb, 21-inch, beautiful baby. I was eager to begin my role as a grandpa. When I shared this news with some of the others at the center, a few of them immediately interpreted the birth of my first grandchild as the reason I was spared – with no permanent damage from the SAH. Philosophically, they said it just wasn't my time. I still had stuff to do here. I was still needed.

In my wanderings to pass the time, I discovered something called a quiet room about half way down a dead end hallway where all other doors were shut. I only visited briefly and I only returned to it one other time during my stay. There was never anyone else around. It was no more than a large walk-in closet but its decor, which included a small organ, left no doubt of its spiritual purpose. There was a sort of guest book where earlier patients and their loved ones had written their individual words of hope and appreciation. I said a quick prayer to the Great Spirit to protect my family and thanked Him for granting me an extension here on earth and for my astounding recovery. I dried a tear and then moved on to see if I would encounter anyone I knew in the busy hallway leading to the kiosk.

Various groups came together for the exercises or sat together at mealtimes. There were also some external activities (like Italian cooking classes or watercolor painting) that patients could sign up for with a small additional fee. I would also meet others at the small, in-house kiosk buying snacks and essentials or even local souvenirs. In this manner, I got to know some of my fellow patients. I was surprised one day to see my former roommate from the stroke unit, the welder.

He was seated outside in the shade on a bench placed along the entrance road and in his right hand he held an escapee from the Marlboro pack now opened and half empty. I was disappointed for him and was foolish enough to think I had found him in time and could encourage him to stop. There he was, a fresh survivor, not badly damaged, still in rehab, smoking - the number two risk factor for stroke victims. Maybe a friendly word of concern was what he needed, so I sat down next to him, upwind, and gestured at his right hand. He just smiled. He knew it himself. I don't understand things like that. It just tells me some things in life are harder to do than surviving a stroke.

The German language has a formal form and an informal form. We really don't have anything like it in the English language. The informal form, which we can think of as being on a first name basis, is generally reserved for long time acquaintances, close friends and family or, perhaps, nowadays among members of the same age group. Among strangers, the formal form is used. Here at the center, all that was suspended and although they came from all over Germany and were of different ages, everyone was immediately known only by their first name – the informal form was used – very unusual from my previous experience in Germany. How easy it was to become part of a conversation with total strangers at this place. The explanation could lie in the subconscious. These light conversations take your mind briefly off of your own problem and, obviously, this was something we all had in common. We were all handicapped; it was new for most of us and it was because of something that went wrong in our heads.

As I learned more about other people's lives, something started to change in my own. My stroke had left me with more understanding. My world was expanded. I discovered I had sympathy for the weaknesses in others. I found that I could simply listen to problems without having the urge to solve them and I threw away my own former, shielded, uninformed judgments. My life experience had not prepared me to solve the kind of stories that were shared here anyway. Most of these, like my own, had no easy solution and by solution, I mean cure. These good people were not admitted to this center as a result of their own choices of action. They had not given up. They were not "copping out" to avoid facing some personal problem. They needed to be here because they had been dealt a bad hand in the game of life. Processes beyond the current state of medical knowledge were operating within their brains and bodies. I showed a sincere interest to understand and be attentive if someone wanted to talk to me about their illness. We were all victims. I knew from my own recent experience that the brain can produce unwanted distractions all by itself and our best machines and doctors are very far from any comprehensive explanation of the mind-body relationship. Everyone one of these patients just wanted to have a normal life back.

Some were stoic about it. Knowing their diagnosis had no cure, they just hoped for some relief or a little more time before the illness incapacitated the next part of their body. Some were frustrated that all the tests and medical equipment failed to identify any physical abnormalities. Their complaint was so real to them and ever present in their minds. They questioned the doctors over and over again seeking some explanation or at least words of hope to hang on to for understanding. They blamed the doctors for not helping them. This attitude was observed by some of the "old timers" who said privately to me, "She is not going to improve if she doesn't relax and stop denying what the doctor tells her. She's not trying."

This a good place to say a few words about trust. A stroke leaves behind a lot of unanswered questions and that's not nice. We have a desire to have all the answers in nice little boxes in just the right places. Certainty equals security. We seek answers to eliminate our fears – the fear that it could happen again without warning or that our disabilities or crying spells may last indefinitely. A lack of trust produces fear, which affects the autonomic nervous system very powerfully and negatively. Fear and worry can make you sick. Trust is a choice when you are thinking of the effects of your stroke. Some people seem to trust easily, some don't. When you don't trust your doctor, it interferes with your treatment plan since the success of that plan depends on your willingness to put into practice the advice you are given. A questioning and mistrusting patient spends more time and energy seeking reassurance from the doctor and others than in actually doing their program. Since compliance inevitably suffers, they usually do not get the results they hope for.

In the next chapter, I relate how trusting your doctor is not always the whole story. Some lingering doubts remain, answers I have not heard, questions that I cannot express. I guess it is like religion. You just have to believe.

G. M. PEACH

"Yesterday is history. Tomorrow is a mystery. And today? Today is a gift. That's why we call it the present."

Babatunde Olatunji

CHAPTER 6

Making sense of things

Is that it? Just luck? Maybe. Or maybe the 'Gods in Green' think a 'mere patient' cannot understand a more intricate answer. At any rate, if you are like me, at some point during your recovery you will feel a need to know more about what happened to you, and then you must seek the answers elsewhere. Author Siri Hustvedt believes intellectual curiosity about one's illness is born of a desire for mastery. In other words, the victim has to want to understand the illness in order to feel well again. So, I set out to discover what had really happened to me.

Such a major threat to life and still, when you ask your doctor to tell you why it happened, chances are you will not receive useful information. What makes a "small defect" burst without warning then seal itself off, remaining undetected by cerebral angiography? In this age of medical breakthroughs and technical advances, doctors still answer questions about stroke with, "We just don't know. A stroke is a mysterious accident." The American bumper sticker "Shit happens!" was probably written by a doctor who didn't know what else to say. My doctors really couldn't explain it. They don't realize at the time that their honest answer is very frustrating for the patient; at least it was for me. In any case, ask why you are left unscarred when the statistics show that others were not so lucky and you will wait in vain for an answer.

This was the "Why me?" factor starting to take effect. Why had this happened to me, someone with no risk factors? Why had I survived the SAH when the statistical odds are against it? Why did the bleeding stop and leave no trace of a burst aneurysm? There must be more to it! How was I to help other stroke victims by simply saying "Wish you luck?" I had been given a gift. I wanted to say thank you and put it to good use.

I am alive and well! Is that a miracle? An intervention by God? That seemed to be what they were telling me and for some people that is enough. Ten weeks have passed since the attack. Not only did I survive a massive bleed and the pain, but I seemed to have no permanent, major cell damage – at least to those cells responsible for mobility and speech. I had made remarkable progress, but I needed to understand what had happened. I needed to "own it" as the motivational speaker would say.

Full recovery to me means coming to terms with

the relevant statistics: The number of non-traumatic red strokes is roughly 10.5 in 100,000 population per year. In the USA alone that is about 30,000 and 75% of those who suffer a subarachnoid hemorrhage never recover. Approximately 14 percent of the survivors have returned or are on the way to leading fairly functional lives. So, I thanked my guardian angel for the present and now I keep putting one word next to the other, one line at a time as I learn more about the mind and the brain.

True, sometimes things seem to happen for no apparent reason: an act of circumstance, an act of God, an act of Nature? When a bad thing happens in our world, they use words like tragedy, catastrophe, and disaster, with adjectives like terrible, unimaginable, and sad. When it is a good thing that happens, where there is hope, people call it lucky. They call it a wonder, a blessing, or a miracle. The thought implied at both ends of this spectrum is that the forces which brought about the illness did so in a way which is outside of the natural course of events. Hearing from other patients that it *just* wasn't my time or being told by the doctors that I was *just* lucky was *just* not enough for me. My progress was *just* too good to be true. There *just* had to be a better explanation. I *just* needed a better understanding. Was I active in achieving this or was it *just* a miracle after all?

At the rehab center, I noticed many miracles all around me, the miracles of everyday life. I noticed the things we take for granted in our immediate surroundings:

the sun coming up over the ridge every morning, the many shades of green in a mixed forest in the summer, the singing of the birds, the long-legged mosquitoes buzzing my room that look so bloodthirsty but don't bite, the giant military transport aircraft able to lift three combat tanks into the air and then fly several hundred feet above a German clinic where every doorway is stenciled with the words "Absolute quiet please!" In my army days, we used to call it "the sound of freedom." You can bet I called it something else from my bed in the clinic. But these are different times and I am getting away from my point.

I remembered a story from the Ripley's *Believe It or Not* book, published around 1970, about a guy named Phineas Gage. He is remembered for surviving an accident in which a crowbar-like tool went right through his skull removing chunks of his brain as it exited. The headline read "The incredible story of Phineas Gage" who in 1848 was a railroad construction worker that worked with explosives to excavate rocks. One day while tamping down the explosive powder, "a spark from the tamping iron ignited the powder, causing the iron to be propelled at high speed straight up through his skull. It entered under the left cheek bone shattering the upper jaw, passing back of the left eye, and exited out through the top of the head," according to the Ludlow Vermont newspaper of the day. He was talking and walking again within minutes. His doctor reported one month later that he was expected to fully recover *"with inconsiderable disturbance of function.*" Talk about being blessed! Neurologists still study his case today.

About the only thing Phineas and I really had in common was the walking and talking so soon after the event. But his story still makes you wonder. Luck is all around. I thank the ambulance drivers and the doctors for their roles in my miracle: the scientists who invented non-invasive diagnostic machines and the pharmacists who figured out a pill that could prevent vasospasms, the experienced nurses we depend on and the therapists who understand mind-body healing. I appreciate the fellow who left the parking space for me at the emergency room entrance that day. I recognize my good fortune in being transferred to a special stroke unit and not sent to a regular hospital intensive unit. I thank my lucky stars for my wife and each member of my family and friends who were there to keep me here, and for having the patience to understand the healing process of stroke victims.

Speaking of my wife, who I am convinced is actually an angel with x-ray vision who can look into my head, encouraged me to use my doctor appointments to discuss the "Why me?" factor, i.e., my feelings. So, at my final appointment with Cap'n Ahab, I asked him the questions: Why did this happen? What caused it? Why is it that there is "inconsiderable disturbance of function" from such a well-known killer? Will it happen again? Is it genetic? I needed answers. As anticipated, he provided all the familiar reassurances and then asked me if these thoughts were a burden to me. I said, "No not really, you have said I will be fine. I have to believe you and continue on with my recovery. I think I am alright with it now." This was not one hundred percent true. I just didn't want to admit then that something was still unnerving to me. After all, I am a tough guy. I would deal with these feelings somehow. At any rate, at least I could now tell my wife that I had discussed it with the doctor. So, no further appointment was made – that is, until the day before my scheduled release, when incredibly, luck entered my story one more time.

It was a warm afternoon by German weather standards, about 90 degrees. I had more "leisure time" on my schedule and decided I would try the walk into the village for an ice cream and some sun at a sidewalk cafe. I noticed a young woman leaving the building from another entrance and as our paths and timing converged at a point in the parking lot, I thought, "Why walk in this heat when I could hitch a ride." I put on my most charming and helpless look and asked her if she could drop me off at the bottom of the hill. She considered it for a moment, saw that I was carrying the water bottle issued to patients and said, "Yes." We only had about three minutes together before reaching the intersection where I was to get out. Can you guess who she was? Can you tell me why she crossed my path that day?

Of course, she was the psychotherapist, the missing link in my recovery plan. As it happened, I was very open about my feelings when she asked me why I was there. Thinking again of my wife's urgings, I asked for and she gave me her name. So the next morning, I was able to schedule a last minute appointment. About an hour after our talk, I checked out of the clinic as planned and the result of that conversation? This book! Let me explain.

During the standard time allocated for an appointment, we talked about my first fear, "Where the hell did it come from and will it happen again?" and, my new question, "Why was my brain not annihilated?" She got me to open up to her about my new emotions and the changes in my sensory inputs, and of course, my eyes watered. Why did that happen every time I tried to talk about my stroke? The medical and care-giving professions had done their jobs. I was alive and well - at least to all outward appearances. Survivors are expected to go back to their lives, like wounded soldiers treated to the point where they are fit enough to return to the front. However, perhaps like some of those soldiers with PTSD, survivors of SAH just can't return to the former innocence they had prior to the attack.

She understood that a stroke has an emotional side to it and she could see what I hide so well. An interesting concept evolved out of this talk: She thought my recovery and future well-being should include "an activity that is free of expectations." For the life of me, I couldn't imagine anything that would meet that criterion.

Then, out of the blue, she concluded, "It will be good for you to write a book." No daily minimums. No deadlines. No expectations. She knew many questions were trapped in my male brain, just as my wife did. Maybe the therapist gives that advice to all stroke victims, or maybe she noticed my eyes tearing as we discussed it. Anyway, she knew that it wasn't important whether I finished the book or not. Regardless of the outcome, it was to be just the slow moving vehicle that allowed me to work through what had happened in my brain.

Remember in Chapter 2, one day in the stroke unit, when I was prevented from sinking too low by the timely appearance of the physical therapist. What I didn't mention in that chapter is the fact that I bawled like a baby when my wife and kids came to visit in that first week. Depression and strange emotions can take hold after a stroke, sometimes during rehab or after you go home. Post-stroke depression is classified as major when it lasts longer than two weeks. Minor may also last longer than two weeks but involves less functional impairment. Mild or major, crying is the most common emotional problem faced by stroke survivors. Crying is an expected coping response. It can be – but not always – caused by physical brain damage from the stroke. Although it may look and feel like depression, there is another, peculiar stroke-induced condition, known as post-stroke laughing/crying (PLC) or "neurologic emotionalism," which is a physical neurologic not a psychologic disorder. It is a secondary occurrence to brain injury and the actual factors which produce it are not well understood. Patients may find themselves crying uncontrollably at something that is pleasant or perhaps only moderately sad. Most people with PLC do not have a diagnosable mood disorder, and many do not manifest any depressive symptoms at all. Estimates of the prevalence of PLC vary from 7% to up to 48.5% of stroke survivors, with a greater prevalence found in inpatient populations and during the acute post-stroke period.

The negative impact of PLC and depression on stroke survivors is well recognized. It is important to distinguish PLC from depression. Both can become chronic and slow down the course of rehabilitation. Again, I was very lucky to have been in a stroke unit where early intervention by healthcare professionals gave me the proper motivation before the distress could become established as a mood disorder. My eyes still get watery sometimes when I talk with people about what happened to me, but time has freed me of those uncontrollable stress tears. I am passed the acute post-stroke period.

Stroke places greater challenges on some people than others. I got off lightly, but strong motivation with the goal of independence after rehabilitation is important for any recovery. Some survivors have more damage to the brain, perhaps because of a delay in getting to the proper care facility. Of course, the severity and the location of the individual stroke may cause some victims to have to work harder and longer than others as they regain various degrees of functionality. Some may be surprised to learn that medical studies show personality type plays a large role in stroke rehabilitation. People who react well to stress, control anxiety, and are generally optimistic about life before a stroke are most likely to react well to life after the stroke, even with some functional loss. The point here is to make sense of what happened and then move on. A positive attitude is the key. Do the exercises. Rise to a new challenge. You can only make it better. Only you can make it better.

Who really knows what powers the mind may have to heal the physical body if given the chance? The US Army that's who! It taught me that "Quitters never win, and winners never quit!" It also taught me the "attitude checks," initially intended to get a group of soldiers into the right mindset for facing an unpleasant task. The troops quickly expanded the verses with typical GI humor. It starts by someone shouting out the first check and others shouting the responses. It goes like this:

ATTITUDE CHECK:	THIS PLACE SUCKS!
Positive attitude check:	This place positively sucks!
Negative attitude check:	No place sucks like this place sucks!
Relative attitude check:	Even my uncle thinks this place sucks!
Airborne attitude check:	This place sucks all the way!

Ranger attitude check:	This place sucks, but it is only a technique!
Marine attitude check:	This place doesn't suck enough!
Air Force attitude check:	That place down there sucks!
Comparative attitude check:	No other place sucks as much as this place sucks!
Historical attitude check:	No place has ever sucked as much as this place sucks!
Predictive attitude check:	No other place will ever suck as much as this place sucks!
Qualitative attitude check:	Even if this place were 100% better it would still suck!
Agricultural attitude check:	This place sucks the root!
Mathematical attitude check:	This place sucks the cube root!
Existential attitude check:	This place exists, therefore it sucks!
Mystical attitude check:	This place sucks the beard of the hairy gnome who dwells in the cave of the four winds!

At some point in your recovery, you might need an attitude check. You see, no matter how you look at it, no one wants to be in a place that sucks! Humor helps you to look at things from a different perspective and not dwell on the negatives. It is, literally, all in your head - an attitude, a state of mind.

It may take a long time to recover to the prestroke levels of functioning, but stick with it – the best chances for getting there are when you start as soon as possible and do not lose any time to depression. In my story, I can honestly say that I never gave myself the option of dying or accepting disability for longer than one second. Accept what happened to you, but you don't ever want to accept permanent disability. I hope you too are lucky enough to have a caregiver who lets you work to your current limits with the goal of overcoming them. My physical therapist jump started my willpower at just the right moment. You may have to think about this in terms of what the Roman philosopher Cicero told Caesar in the year 45 BC: "It is far better to wear out than rust out."

~~~~~~~~~~~~~~~~

Just when you think everything is clear… Remember I told you about the exit interview? Well, I left out this part. I mentioned to the doctor that I was still experiencing strange headaches. This is when Cap'n Ahab explained to me, "You are not the same person you were before. There are two parts to your new feelings: the neurological and the psychological. The source of your headache now is no longer neurologic. It may be a memory of what happened to you." I said to myself, What the *!#x? Was he saying that my mind was somehow reminding my body of the painful pressure that was no longer there? Bingo! Well, my search for answers about my stroke had just been served another portion of carrot salad. This was another challenge to my understanding and something else I needed to explore.

Bear with me now as this gets a bit technical regarding this "memorized" headache. It is an area of leading edge brain research. In reality, the nervous system remembers any experience that overwhelms it. A life altering moment activates the self-protective limbic-hypothalamic system that acts to secrete chemicals that interfere with our perception of high-charged emotion until we are ready to deal with it.

The limbic system is a set of primitive brain structures called the "old mammalian brain" located on top of the brainstem. It goes about its ancient agenda interpreting and controlling various emotional responses, storing memories, and regulating hormones. Two large limbic system structures, the amygdala and hippocampus play important roles in memory. The amygdala is considered the brain's primary emotional center and communicates with all other sensory input systems through extensive neural communications channels. Emotions assist in deciding what needs attention, which impacts what we ultimately remember. What memories are stored and where the memories are stored is determined in this system. Any stressful or overwhelming event is encoded and stored in one of two places: the "explicit" and the "implicit" memory.

The explicit memory is conscious and enables us to make sense of what happened and is stored in the nerve centers of the body. The implicit memory is encoded in emotional and sensory recall in the subconscious. Research suggests this determination is based on how huge an emotional response an event invokes. Experiences that are emotionally too overwhelming to deal with are stored somatically, as a body memory. Thereafter, they are expressed as an unconscious response to stress.

The limbic system is the interface between our emotional states and the stored memories of physical stimuli. In other words, what we don't remember with our minds, we remember with our bodies, our hearts, our 'guts' (the visceral nervous system). Your thoughts and the way you perceive situations are actually written into your muscles, sinew and viscera - every cell of your body. Not one of our experiences is lost to us. Something that 'reminds' our brains of an emotional situation - a smell, a song, a person that looks like someone from our past – triggers an automatic, self-protective 'freeze-frame' response. This reflexive reaction occurs too quickly; before the information reaches the cortex where it can be evaluated rationally. Walking is a good example: You don't remember learning to walk but, years later, each foot plays its part perfectly. No rational thinking is necessary. Every cell in your body "thinks." Some of the most pivotal lessons in human survival are learned at a time that our bodies, but not our minds, can remember.

At every moment of your life, your body is thinking for you. It remembers. Time doesn't heal wounds, it conserves them. In order to heal from a body memory, you need to let your body release the memory. After you release them, your body no longer feels the need to experience them. Releasing a body memory is not fun. You must surrender to the awful pain or feelings and allow your body to re-feel really badly for a little while. However, you have already survived the pain, so you can survive the memory. YOU ARE WHAT YOU THINK!

It all sounds pretty complicated to me, but after having a stroke it couldn't hurt to have every cell start thinking "full recovery" every waking minute. I found that my mammalian memory could do more than give me a headache. My stroke had a disorienting effect by distorting my sensory inputs and I still feel "slowed down." Feeling tired is a common complaint after a stroke. About 30-70% of survivors suffer from fatigue. It can be frustrating and can slow down recovery. It can even affect those who are doing well after stroke. After the experience of a stroke, it takes some time to regain your self-confidence. It seems the old, ordered self remembers what happened to it and still thinks it must be hurt. Having a stroke is a very frightening experience. Like any unexpected illness it can put you face to face with death and turn your world upside down. After such a shock, the mind needs time to learn that the brain has recovered. Whereas in the early weeks following the stroke the mind can control the healing process, at this stage, the body has to provide feedback and tell the mind that it is OK. The cells have to relearn or remember what their healthy state was like prior to the event. I had recovered all of my functionalities, yet I still had poor endurance and was cautious about exertion. And, why was I unable to concentrate on anything for longer than an hour?

Disturbances of the visceral nervous system are common in stroke patients, with blood pressure regulation being the most common problem. The visceral nervous system jumps into action immediately, but it is very slow to shut down and allow the body to return back from the emergency status. Once your stress response has been activated, the system wisely remembers it and keeps you in a state of readiness. The unconscious memories are still stimulating the mind, trying to insure it has the time it needs to heal the brain. It seems the mind first gets the brain and everything else working, then it can start healing itself – and, that takes time. Concentrating on work and exerting yourself are not relaxation and the mind cannot take care of itself for it is doing all the other things you ask of it. So, now you know the long version of Cap'n Ahab's explanation of my lingering headache.

The National Stroke Association has compiled a list of ideas that can help:

- Know that fatigue is a genuine symptom after stroke; you will tire more easily.
- Don't overdo it. It will take time to build your endurance. Plan rest time.

- Find out what exercises, foods or habits can help restore your strength.
- Try not to spend too much time in bed. Bed rest can result in loss of muscle strength.
- The sudden change in blood pressure when you stand up can make you dizzy. Be sure to stand up or get out of bed slowly.

Both the survivor and the caregiver have to take the time to accept what has happened. Accept your new feelings (the new reality) as they come to you – take baby steps, and trust that time will help you. I was beginning to trust in what "Cap'n Ahab" had said and, as things turned out, the expert knew what he was talking about: The brain (or the mind) will gradually begin to see that everything is fine and those memories will begin to fade away, along with the headaches. You can be confident of this.

As explained to me, even though it was never located, I must have had a faulty blood vessel at birth that did its job well for 56 years. Then, after years of borderline high pressure, the vessel burst and blood flowed out into the fluid spaces surrounding the brain and caused pressure on the cells in that area of my brain – pretty simple. It could have happened at age 26 or 76 and they assure me there is very little chance that it will happen again. I guess William Shakespeare said it best, "Such as we are made of, such we be."

I take comfort now in the fact that I have been

examined inside and out: I take my daily dosage of effective pills and I know the risk factors and the symptoms. When I asked the doctor about my lingering fears, he answered very seriously, "You can die from many things, but not this, not anymore." Seems he was right again! I end this chapter with the acceptance that I was involved in a dangerous incident, the affirmation that I have recovered, and with extreme relief that I have test results that reveal nothing to cause me further fear. Today is a gift. But, the journey is not over when the victim returns home.

LUCKY STROKE

"The winds of God are always blowing, but you must set the sails."

Unknown

G. M. PEACH

CHAPTER 7

Time to go home

Spain beat the Netherlands to win the World Cup for the first time ever. The German soccer team clinched a third place and life in Europe would return to normal once again for at least the next four years. BP got their deep sea oil leak plugged after 86 days and 5 million barrels had gushed into the marine waters of the Gulf leaving an ecological effect that will be around for the rest of my lifetime. Schools have re-opened and autumn is just around the corner. As valuable as it was, there was nothing more I was going to learn at the rehab center. It was time for me to get out of there – besides, one more dish of carrot salad would have killed me.

My stroke is now for me alone. My wife doesn't have to install ramps around the house for a wheelchair or prepare non-chew foods to nourish me. No one can learn what a stroke does by looking at me. No cognitive or physical consequences to my stroke are apparent, other than the semi-permanent mild headache. How do you explain to others that only the invisible problems remain? In the case of diffused bleeding in the brain, these can be the cause for frustration and upset: disoriented senses, difficulty concentrating, short-term memory lapses, weakness, slow responses, egocentric behavior, reduced inhibition, and general impatience towards interruptions. These are the battle scars stroke recovery can leave behind.

Every once in a while, I have to stop working and lie down for 15-20 minutes. At a gathering with friends I may get dizzy and have to sit down or lean against a wall so they won't know. Maybe my speech appears too deliberate, (i.e., slow) and there is still some tearing when I think about what has happened or about the others back at the rehab center. I am different too now in crowds, they are too overwhelming. I used to have my "radar" on all the time. I checked out all the new images around me to see everyone and everything. My reactions were faster. Now I no longer notice the full surroundings; my senses just pick up the immediate inputs. It is as if I have only enough energy to focus on just one stimulus, sort of like a wide tunnel vision. I miss a lot of what is happening on the peripheries. I still have to mute the TV or radio to talk with someone. Sometimes, I yearn for the quiet of the rehab center where you go into the woods and pause on the trail with your eyes closed to hear all the various sounds, from near and far, that are within range.

What remains are the lucky scars, the little 'bumps' I sometimes feel just under the surface. These aren't the kind of deficits a stranger would notice in a short conversation. But family and friends are aware that something is off. Simple connections seem to misfire, for example, sometimes I misstate the obvious when speaking. I often say a related word or one that starts with the same letter in place of the intended word, but I immediately catch it and quickly insert the correct word. The medical term for this is apraxia of speech (AOS). I have also shocked friends with my outbursts of swearing at other drivers while driving in heavy traffic and I have too easily lost patience with loved ones in what was a stressful situation only to me. It just takes time. These residual effects are always with me now as I move on with my life, but I think these too are slowly fading away and I confidently hope that these invisible problems will also disappear with the passage of time as the cells of my mammalian brain get themselves reoriented to less traumatic times. But, like all survivors, I still wanted to find some reasonable explanation for why it happened to me.

Now I'm lucky to be reestablishing contact to friends. Through the smiles and the eyes – I am pleased to hear "You don't look like you've had a stroke." I really don't want to contradict them on this point. I am extremely lucky in this regard and happy that there is no visible proof of this attack. My stroke affected the brain and the brain is located inside the skull. Who can say what that is supposed to look like on the outside? They probably have the stereotype survivor in mind, the one who, at least during some part of the recovery phase, presents a noticeable droop in the eyelid or a lopsided facial expression or a heavy limb that just won't respond. They prepare to visit the survivor as if there is a contagious disease hovering about or, at the other extreme; they come prepared to offer too much sympathy and sorrow for the victim. I guess it is just part of the general fear of the word stroke. There is a misconception that everyone who survives a stroke will be left with a permanent and visible handicap. People think, "It must not have been a stroke. If you are not handicapped, then you didn't have one." In general, people know so little about a stroke.

It is rare to meet with people who go beyond the "how are you doing?" question. Some people are scared or curious enough to actually want to understand the details about what happened to me. What was to blame for the attack; what symptoms did I have leading up to the brain attack? These are questions we all, especially the survivor, want to have answered.

I am one of the victims who will never know for sure what was to blame for the SAH. None of the standard FAST warning signs (Face, Arms, Speech, and Time) applied to me. Just the crippling headache that came out of nowhere. Most instances of SAH in our world today are attributed to lifestyle exposures and that does account for a great percentage of the statistics. Truthfully, I have never smoked or snorted anything and my alcohol intake is always in moderation. With age, my blood pressure rose a bit, but was normally only borderline high at 150/90 (although it had been that way for a while). Although, all of us have to live with some forms of stress – familial, financial, marital, employment, health, etc. I lead a fairly relaxed and manageable life. My motto was not so much "Don't worry. Be happy," but rather, as Baz Luhrmann said, "Don't worry. The real troubles in your life are apt to be things that never crossed your worried mind, the kind that blindside you at 4 pm on some idle Tuesday."

Most survivors will not be able to avoid one anxiety, especially, in the first six months. Even now, after more than a year, the fear of a second stroke is never far from me. The first one appeared out of nowhere. A vessel exploded in my brain and nothing has really been done about it. It was like getting a cut and giving it time to scab over and heal. He couldn't even put a band aid on it. Will it happen again? Studies show that 25 percent of those who recover from their first stroke will have another stroke within 5 years. For me, nothing was found and repaired. I wondered, "How strong is my self-repair? How long will it hold?" Of course, I still wonder: are the 25 percent of those who have a second episode cases like mine? The patients that have an aneurysm identified and surgically repaired have a different set of risks when moving on with their recovery. The commonly available information is not broken down to this level of detail.

Victims have a need to know the cause of the ordeal they have just survived and will grab most any straw to find it. What had been explained to me as unexplainable in my doctor-patient conversations was still unexplained and that gnawed at me. If, as they say, half the risk of stroke remains unexplained by conventional risk factors, then that half must be attributed to the unconventional factors, right? My recovery was likened to forces outside the natural course of events. So why not the cause too? I decided to look up some of these other "unconventional" risk factors.

In the weeks leading up to the hemorrhage I had a craving for pepper. I couldn't get enough pepper. I had not used a pepper shaker more than ten times in my entire life and now, all I wanted was pepper. I wanted it all the time. I started putting the pepper shaker on the dining table and used it at every meal – a lot – on everything, no matter what was served. Even spicy foods tasted good to me now. In talking with some friends about what happened to me, I have learned something interesting: pepper is an herb known to have medicinal properties. Pepper is used, among other things, to stimulate blood circulation, brain functions, and lower the blood pressure. Don't take this as medical advice, but the therapeutic effect of pepper is well proven in lowering high blood pressure. Cayenne pepper, in particular, aids the body to balance pressure levels and resist abnormal bleeding. Listen to your body when it is trying to tell you something. A new craving may be something to ask your doctor about.

I noticed only one other strange thing in the months preceding my stroke that may or may not have been a warning sign or even related to it. Maybe it is not worth mentioning, but the only other unusual physical sensation I had were the two or three times when I experienced chills at night causing me to shiver uncontrollably. Lying in bed under the blanket, my teeth were chattering and my knees were shaking for a few seconds almost like minor convulsions. The whole episode lasted no more than one to two minutes and causing me some momentary concern then went away fairly quickly and I had a good night's sleep. There were several weeks in between these episodes and no other symptoms, I didn't worry about it. Now I am curious about what caused this and if, perhaps an infection had some relationship to the SAH.

A 2010 study suggests that an association between weather and stroke is virtually non-existent. Thus, seasonal associations between weather and stroke proved to be only a popular misconception. Is there a link between the lunar phases and medically unexplained stroke? According to the University of Glasgow Medical School, there is a statistically significant association between admission to the acute stroke unit and the full moon phase. Well, there wasn't a full moon on the day of my stroke. Next? My personal favorite is that I was bombarded with a stray beam from the US government's top secret high energy auroral radiation program (HAARP), a ground penetrating radar beam that is bounced off the atmosphere back into the ground to look for underground bunkers on the other side of the world, which arrived at just the right angle to split open one of by brain's blood vessels as it passed by at a speed faster than light. Less far-fetched, perhaps the most likely causal relationship can be found some physical predisposition of the individual.

My brother immediately feared that the cause of my stroke was somehow hereditary because he remembered our grandmother had two siblings who had survived strokes (though we didn't know what kind). Although familial preponderance suggests a genetic influence in the occurrence of stroke, studies of this connection have failed to identify markers and are inconclusive. I think he was relieved when I was able to tell him that no definite links have been found.

The completion of the "Human Genome Project" in 2005 has indeed improved our knowledge about the potential role of genetics in complex disorders, including stroke. Scientists at the Herlev University Clinic, in Copenhagen, Denmark claim to have found a gene that increases a person's chances of having a stroke. They claim it is actually a defect in the HFE gene and one of the most common inheritable genetic defects, especially in Europe. The gene is associated with the regulation of iron at a cellular level, but why this gene appears to cause an increased risk of stroke is still undetermined.

At Harvard, a team of researchers think they have a gene that carries instructions for making a hormone that can lower the risk of stroke. Their research suggests a mutation in a gene that affects blood vessel function can lead to a failure to produce a certain hormone and logically, this mutation should be much more common in people who experience stroke. Meanwhile, a team in Germany together with Dutch researchers has discovered an enzyme that is responsible for the death of nerve cells after a stroke. An experimental new drug dramatically reduces brain damage and preserves brain functions in mice, even when given hours after the stroke. The identification of an enzyme with a key role in killing nerve cells after stroke in mice currently makes inhibition of this enzyme in humans the most promising new therapeutic approach in this often deadly or disabling illness.

The search continues, but preventive genetic testing and preventive cures are a long way off. The identification of genes that contribute to stroke could help to diagnose and determine who is at greater risk and suggest lifestyle modifications to the risk population or develop new individualized medicines to reduce the overall risk of stroke in the future. Further research and the benefits of gene therapy could significantly reduce the death and disability from stroke, but universal testing and the protective drug for stroke remain elusive. Until that day arrives, we must rely on the conventional risk factors and, yes, on miracles and luck.

~~~~~~~~~~~~~~~~

As researchers continue to zero in on the hormones and the stroke gene, other scientists are busy searching for the "luck gene." In the same way the onset of stroke varies, so does the aftermath of stroke. Some victims experience a complete recovery and others endure permanent and severe disability, although most survivors will recover some functional independence with time. Why is this so? What explains the differences? What if the lucky 'gene' is just something in the mind of the survivor - not in the brain or the body to be found by genetic engineers - but rather by shamans in the spirit?

There is a story recounted by New York hand surgeon Kenneth Kamler that happened on his trip as the expedition doctor in the Himalayas. He witnessed an extraordinary event on Mount Everest. Although technically not a stroke, this relates a traumatic brain hemorrhage: A sherpa named Pasan was crossing a steep divide on a ladder when he had a terrible accident. "He fell head first into a crevasse about, about 80 feet down, and landed head first, and he was sort of wedged down there, refrigerated, in this crevasse for about half an hour before he could be pulled out," Kamler said. Pasan was unconscious and his health deteriorated quickly – his face and eyelids were bloated, his blood pressure dropped and his pupils stopped responding to light. Kamler knew his brain was bleeding and there was no way he could possibly live till morning. Kamler watched helplessly as Pasan was surely slipping away. But then a group of sherpas in the medical tent made a circle around Pasan and they started to chant. Kamler described it as "a deep, low droning sound that seemed to emanate from within the mountain itself. The chanting continued through the night, and Pasan's pulse grew stronger. "I very much felt like if the chanting stopped, my patient would die. I felt like he was living through that, that chanting. That was keeping him alive," Kamler continued. "After a while, his pupils started to react again. At dawn, the chanting stopped, and Pasan was able to speak. He had really turned a corner, and I can't explain this in any medical way." Dr. Kamler's baffled summary of that case sounded a lot like what my doctor had told me. Pasan was simply "one, lucky S.O.B."

Throughout this book I mention many events that happened and that I interpreted as lucky. Personality type appears to play a large role in stroke rehabilitation. People who are generally optimistic about life before a stroke are most likely to react well to life after the stroke. I have always considered myself to be lucky and in researching this aspect of my stroke, I found many sources that deal with the concept.

Azriela Jaffe, author of "Create Your Own Luck," for example, attributes luck to toxic-free thinking. Negative beliefs prevent you from seeing the solution to your problems, she suggests. Opening your mind allows you to move beyond the obstacle by finding your way around it. Toshu Fukami, a highly successful Japanese businessman, wrote "Lucky Fortune" to explain the whys and wherefores of his success and makes a similar association between good fortune and positive thinking. Lucky people, he says, are those who have a knack for finding something to their advantage in any given situation. Both writers define luck as a state of mind, an attitude (which reminds me of the Army's time tested method shared in the last chapter).

A very important part of stroke recovery involves the survivor's own ability to adapt and the will to recover. Numerous studies have confirmed evidence that a small number of lucky people carry a gene which helps to protect them against the damaging effects of cell loss from disease and aging. Research indicates carriers of a certain form of the 5-HTTLPR gene have difficulty disengaging attention from emotional stimuli and are more at risk compared to people who have a different form of the gene. Much has been written about the "resilience" gene.

Resilience researcher Ann Masten describes the resilience gene – and the complex interplay in some people between genes, environment, and health – as something that sparks and sustains what she calls "ordinary magic." The evidence collected to date shows that overcoming adversity in life may be easier when some common resilience factors are in place –

fundamental protective systems that work to give people an impressive capacity to adapt when faced with extreme threats. This can be greatly aided through the protection of family looking out for them; a moral compass that guides them and provides self-control and emotional regulation; faith and motivation to master problems; effective teachers and role models; having opportunities to experience the hopes and rewards of doing something that changes what is happening; and, an environment that supports these systems.

Though these are not genes at all, I was also lucky that many of these systems were present in my life at the time of my stroke, for example, a caring family, an effective physical therapist, and a positive belief about the self, also referred to as realistic optimism. Maybe these resilience researchers are on to something. Who can say?

Medical science is not able to answer all the questions. The topics neuroplasticity, body memory, gene research, and resilience are included not because they are some of the hot areas of stroke research, but because they are topics that get the reader thinking about the deepest places within us. The truth is I had been seriously wounded and the effects could have been so much more devastating. Caring family or friends can be one of the most important factors in successful rehabilitation, but the best way to help is actually by helping the patient to get in touch with the source of inner strength – something only the patient can and must do and that is the subject of the next few pages.

~~~~~~~~~~~~~~~~

Ordinarily, it would not be a piece of luck to experience SAH. The popular conception of stroke is anything but positive. But to survive such a stroke and then discover a new awareness of life could well be some good luck. Surviving this major life event teaches us to slow down and appreciate living now.

Why is it that so many stroke survivors say they became a different person after their stroke? In writing about the effects of his stroke, Kirk Douglas says the stroke "changed me into a different person – a person whom I like." He was referring to life's lesson that it is better to give than to receive. Emotional changes are highly frequent in stroke survivors, as Mr. Douglas tells us. How can this be explained? What changes? Why did Cap'n Ahab tell me to my face that I was no longer the same person? Why is the survival and recovery experience – almost without exception – reported to be a change for the positive?

I have written in the previous chapter that a stroke is an emotional experience and that the part of the brain that deals with emotion are the primitive structures located at the top of the brainstem – the limbic system, the "Houston Control" of emotional responses. This area is very close to the tip of the basilar artery, the most common location for subarachnoid hemorrhagic stroke.

Now it appears to researchers that this region is also the origin of altruistic, unselfish behavior. Some say compassion. This works for me. I find that I try to take time to listen to others now.

A number of theories have been postulated to explain how this group of organs functions, which, among other things, control memory and hormonal release. Another stroke victim, Dr. Jill Bolte Taylor, is also a professional neural anatomist. She says she has been positively changed by her stroke experience. In writing about her stroke, she now considers herself "110% functional" but like Douglas, different than before her stroke. "In every way, I have recovered, but I have not returned to being the same person I was before," she says. "Before the stroke, I was much more 'me' oriented, much more career oriented," Taylor says. "And now, I'm not like that anymore. Now, I'm much more about 'we.' I try to use the time that I have here to use my gift to make a positive contribution to how we live our lives and for the health and well-being of other people who are in the place that I have been."

Taylor calls the process "stepping to the right," or shifting to her brain's right hemisphere and the inner peace she experienced during her stroke. This is where we experience the pure immediate, the present. Her left hemisphere, she explains, is where she becomes a single individual, separated from the flowing energy of the universe and concerned only about the detail in her own life and her future. Her stroke shut down this side and she felt as if she was part of much greater whole. Taylor says she can consciously focus her mind on the emotional information presently coming in through her sensory connections, and intercept it before it is assessed and evaluated by the left hemisphere for past and future significance. She believes that if we take the time to use the power circuitry of our right hemisphere, we will project peace into the world and our planet will become more peaceful. It's a legacy from her stroke that Taylor says can work for anyone. Dr. Taylor never used the word compassion, but that is what she is proposing for us all.

Kirk Douglas concluded after his recovery that he had led a fairly selfish life – "dropping friends along the way like barnacles on the keel of a fast moving ship," – just the opposite of altruistic. He wrote that his stroke taught him to be more compassionate, to value friendships more, to be aware of the greater world around him, and to slow down. There is a common thread that runs through the reports of survivors. SAH survivor blogs identify it: "I show my emotions much more now that I used to," and "I have never had so much awareness of life than I have had since this event." It is interesting to me that these two stroke survivors attribute their new outlook on life to the experience of having had a stroke. But their experience with other victims at the time of their recovery is not mentioned. For me, this time during the recovery and rehab phases was really what changed me. Dr. Taylor believes that following a stroke in the left side, the right hemisphere seems to get a bigger share of the vote in how we view our world. I think Dr. Taylor would agree in any case that this new found awareness and compassion for others – no matter which side of the brain produced it – is a real part of the miracle. I am lucky that I now have the ability to appreciate these miracles.

Most of all it is a humbling experience. Now, like Douglas, I appreciate more the selfless service of others and the meaning of friendships. I am fortunate to be able to work again and my family is fine. My stroke has taught me the word "compassion." I find that I have time now for the things which didn't fit into my life before. I took the time to return to the stroke unit to thank the nurses and doctors. They were surprised and happy to see me and they told me that they very rarely get any feedback after a patient leaves their ward. The real benefit comes in changing how you experience the world. Look for things to be grateful for, and you'll start seeing them.

Talking to strangers about myself has never been my thing, but the psychotherapist was right. Just this week, as I put the finishing touches to this book, my wife noticed I can talk about my memories now for the first time without my eyes watering. Without the pain, this book would never have been written. Without the understanding I have gained from writing about my experience, I might not have recovered as completely.

So, now you know "what I did last summer." My story included the technology and the emotions, the machines, the people, and the questions that accompanied me on that long journey back from the twilight zone. While I was away, I learned the importance of time and compassion in the healing process. Life needs more of these two things. I had a lucky stroke and learned from it.

Miracles are all around us. You just need time to see them. I hope you are taking the time. Good luck!

"Even the stones placed in our path can be used
to build something beautiful!"

(*"Auch aus den Steinen, die einem in den Weg gelegt
werden, kann man Schönes bauen!"*)

Goethe

G. M. PEACH

Index

ABOUT THE AUTHOR

Glenn Marshall Peach grew up in the suburbs of Boston and graduated from the United States Military Academy. Now a self-employed business owner and university lecturer, he has fully recovered from the SAH stroke that attacked his brain in 2010. Glenn resides in southern Germany with his wife of 35 years, Gerda Maria.

45250542R00078

Made in the USA
Middletown, DE
28 June 2017